Managing Challenging Patients and Families in Health Care Settings

Eileen Raynor
Editor

Managing Challenging Patients and Families in Health Care Settings

Springer

Editor
Eileen Raynor
Head and Neck Surgery
& Communication Sciences
Duke University Health
Durham, NC, USA

ISBN 978-3-032-10491-5 ISBN 978-3-032-10492-2 (eBook)
https://doi.org/10.1007/978-3-032-10492-2

This Springer imprint is published by the registered company Springer Nature Switzerland AG
The registered company address is: Gewerbestrasse 11, 6330 Cham, Switzerland

Preface

In the dynamic and complex world of healthcare, professionals are continually navigating an array of challenging patient scenarios that test their skills, compassion, and judgment. This book offers a vital exploration of some of the most intricate and often overlooked issues faced by healthcare providers today. Through these pages, readers will gain valuable insights into the multifaceted nature of patient interactions, encompassing language barriers, diverse personality types, custody issues, ethical dilemmas, health literacy challenges, cultural considerations, and communication hurdles. The chapters will help provide guidance on dealing with difficult situations involving minors and patients from different cultures and backgrounds. Included are clinical scenarios that come from real clinical situations healthcare providers face on a regular basis. Information on where to find appropriate resources and best practices is also a central theme throughout the text.

At the core of effective healthcare delivery lies the ability to listen actively and communicate openly. Active listening goes beyond merely hearing words; it involves fully concentrating on the patient, understanding their concerns, and responding thoughtfully. When healthcare providers listen with empathy and without judgment, patients feel valued and understood, which fosters trust and promotes more accurate disclosures. Open communication encourages a two-way dialogue where patients feel safe to express their fears, preferences, and expectations. This open communication can be stressed when patients or their families are upset, apprehensive or defensive and when the providers are having time constraints or numerous "little fires" occurring at the same time vying for attention.

Equally important is body language and messaging. Nonverbal cues—such as eye contact, facial expressions, posture, and gestures—play a crucial role in conveying attentiveness, empathy, and reassurance. When body language aligns with verbal communication, it reinforces trust and helps bridge language or cultural gaps. Conversely, incongruent messages through body language can lead to misunderstandings or feelings of alienation. Taking a deep breath, sitting down, and being present in the moment are important ways to allow for attention to one's own emotional state and consequently, how they are communicating both verbally and nonverbally.

Each chapter in this book delves into real-world scenarios, providing not only a thorough understanding of these challenges but also practical strategies and thoughtful approaches to address them effectively. The ultimate goal is to foster greater awareness, empathy, and competence among healthcare professionals as they strive to deliver equitable and respectful care to all patients, regardless of situation. Keeping the patient at the center of their care will serve as a constant despite external influences. Remembering that there are options and resources to help de-escalate emotional situations or understand cultural and language differences and calling in reinforcements when needed will decrease the overall anxiety that these situations can induce.

Success in healthcare extends beyond clinical expertise; it requires cultural sensitivity, ethical clarity, and exceptional communication skills. This book aims to serve as a guide and a reminder of the profound impact that active listening, open dialogue, and conscious body language can have on patient outcomes and satisfaction. It has been shown in numerous cases that communication or lack thereof is the number one reason for either patient satisfaction with their care and experience or sadly, malpractice claims.

May this resource inspire healthcare providers to approach every challenge with confidence, compassion, and a commitment to excellence.

Durham, NC, USA Eileen Raynor

Acknowledgments

Thank you to all my chapter authors for their excellent contributions. Thank you to my patients, their families, and the many other countless patients who run into difficulty with the healthcare system as it currently is. Thank you to our child life team, our social work team, our medical interpreters, and the many other healthcare team members that make our work easier and improve communication and patient interactions every day.

Most of all, thank you to our tireless, selfless healthcare work force. Without your dedication and commitment, our society would be in a far less safe, caring, and healthy environment. Please remember you are appreciated and vitally important.

Contents

Contributors

Ana-Maria Fernandez Duke Pediatric Plastic and Oral Maxillofacial Surgery, Durham, NC, USA

Ashley Milinichik Patient Navigator, Duke University Hospital, Durham, NC, USA

Monica Ogunsusi Department of Head and Neck Surgery & Communication Sciences, Duke University, Durham, NC, USA

Somtochi Okafor, MD Department of Head and Neck Surgery, Duke University School of Medicine, Durham, NC, USA

Eileen Raynor Head and Neck Surgery & Communication Sciences, Duke University Health, Durham, NC, USA

Shelia Rittgers Duke University Health System, Durham, NC, USA

Yolanda Troublefield Private Practice, Dartmouth, MA, USA

Chelsea Walsh Duke Children's Hospital and Health Center, Durham, NC, USA

Definitions and Descriptions of Personality Types

1

Monica Ogunsusi

Introduction

Child psychology is a branch of psychology that focuses on the emotional, social, behavioral, and cognitive development of infants, children, and adolescents. Across the various developmental stages described in child psychology, a child's personality takes shape. Personality describes the unique interrelation of an individual's emotions, thoughts, and behaviors and how these influence one's interactions with themselves and the world around them. A child's personality is shaped by both inherent traits, such as genetics, and environmental factors, such as culture and life experiences [1, 2].

A fundamental component of personality is **temperament**, which describes a person's emotional disposition, motor activity, reactivity, and self-regulation patterns [1]. Temperament is believed to be a relatively stable trait by many psychologists, with a strong genetic basis [3]. This innate disposition toward a child's internal experience and external environment serves as the foundation for their developing personality.

M. Ogunsusi (✉)
Department of Head and Neck Surgery & Communication Sciences, Duke University, Durham, NC, USA
e-mail: Monica.Ogunsusi@duke.edu

E. Raynor (ed.), *Managing Challenging Patients and Families in Health Care Settings*, https://doi.org/10.1007/978-3-032-10492-2_1

Temperament

In the 1970s, child psychiatrist and researchers Alexander Thomas and Stella Chess developed a classification system to describe the temperaments of children [1]. They identified nine traits that influence a child's temperament. These traits are activity level, rhythmicity, approach and withdrawal, adaptability, intensity of reaction, attention span, threshold of responsiveness, and quality of mood [1, 4]:

- **Activity level:** The level of physical activity a child displays performing daily activities. A child with a high activity level is energetic and looking for ways to explore their environment. Low-activity-level children tend to be still and move slower in pace.
- **Rhythmicity:** Refers to the predictability of basic biological functions such as sleep habits, regularity of bowel functions, and eating habits. Children with high rhythmicity tend to have a dependable schedule for these functions, whereas children with low rhythmicity display more irregular and unpredictable patterns.
- **Approach and withdrawal:** Describes how a child interacts with a new stimuli such as unfamiliar foods, people, or environments. One child may readily approach new stimuli with curiosity and little hesitation, while another may withdrawal, exercise more caution, or take longer to adjust or accept change.
- **Adaptability**: A child's ability to adjust to a new situation.
- **Intensity of reaction**: The energy level with which a child responds to a situation, whether positive or negative. One child may respond to a broken toy with mild, short-lived upset, while another child may experience intense and prolonged sadness.
- **Attention span**: The ability to concentrate on a task, independent of distractions.
- **Distractibility:** How easily distracted from a task a child can be by a stimulus.

- **Threshold of responsiveness:** Refers to the level of sensory stimulation required to elicit a response from a child. Children with low thresholds respond to the slightest change in stimulation, whereas those with higher thresholds require intense or sustained stimuli before responding.
- **Quality of mood**: How positive or negative a child's words, thoughts, and behaviors tend to be.

Recognizing these different characteristics can assist the clinician with their approach to the child and family during a medical encounter, when anxiety is often heightened. Maintaining situational awareness or taking the "temperature of the room" is essential to fostering productive interactions with the patient and their caregivers. Utilization of external resources such as child life specialists or other family members can help reduce anxiety and distractions, allowing care to be delivered at the highest quality. With these nine characteristics identified, Thomas and Chess postulated three general categories of temperament: easy, difficult, and slow to warm up [4, 5].

Easy

The **"easy" child** is characterized by regular routines (such as sleep/wake, eating), is not easily distracted, concentrates on given tasks, is adaptable, curious, and is interested in new things. Their activity levels, threshold of responsiveness, and intensity of reactions are considered mild to moderate in quality. These children generally have a positive affect. Children in this category are thought to be resilient [4, 5].

Difficult

The **"difficult" child** is characterized by more irregular pattern in their physiologic routines. They tend to be easily distracted, have trouble adapting to unexpected events, and withdraw from new people and environments. Their activity levels are high and can be seen as hyperactive and restless. Their mood is labile, as they are typically more sensitive to stimuli and experience their emotions intensely, with a tendency toward negative thoughts and emotions. It can be difficult to soothe these children. These children may require more time to reset and calm down during clinical encounters[4, 5].

Slow to Warm Up

The **"slow-to-warm-up" child** demonstrates variablity in rhythmicity, sensitivity threshold, attention span, and distractibility. The hallmark for a slow-to-warm-up child is their slow adaptability to change and withdrawal from new stimuli, though these children eventually warm up with time. The intensity of their emotions tends to be mild, similar to their activity levels which are low to moderate. Their overall mood tends to lean more towards negative than positive [4, 5]. These children may initially appear "shy" and require time to feel comfortable engaging with the clinician. Purposeful engagement and consistent attention can help facilitate the child's participation.

These categories, though broad, offer a way for parents, caregivers, educators, and providers to understand a child's tendencies and help predict what may or may not be helpful and effective methods to address certain behaviors.

Personality Traits

While temperament describes inherent traits and a person's disposition, personality encompasses a broader set of influences beyond biological factors. As a child develops cognitively and emotionally, temperament evolves into more enduring personality traits that stabilize throughout childhood and adolescence [2].

Psychologists over the past century have identified and organized numerous personality traits through observation and various experimental studies and determined that personality can be described using five characteristics [6, 7]. The five unique factors, sometimes labeled as the **"Big Five," "OCEAN model," "CANOE model,"** or **"five-factor model of personality,"** are as follows: openness, conscientiousness, extroversion, agreeable, and neuroticism [6, 7].

Openness

This trait encompasses imagination, creativity, and a willingness to try new things and experiences [8]:

- **High openness:** Individuals are often imaginative and curious and enjoy intellectual pursuits.
- **Low openness:** Individuals tend to be more practical, prefer routine, and may be less open to new ideas.

Conscientiousness

This trait reflects a person's level of goal orientation, persistence, and organization [8]:

- **High conscientiousness:** Individuals are often organized, responsible, and detail oriented.
- **Low conscientiousness:** Individuals may be more impulsive and less organized and struggle with long-term goals.

Extraversion

This trait describes a person's preference for social interaction and stimulation from the outside world [8]:

- **High extraversion:** Individuals are often sociable and outgoing and enjoy being around people.
- **Low extraversion:** Individuals tend to be more introverted, preferring solitude and quiet reflection.

Agreeableness

This trait reflects a person's tendency to prioritize the needs of others and be cooperative and empathetic [8]:

- **High agreeableness:** Individuals are often kind, compassionate, friendly, and cooperative.
- **Low agreeableness:** Individuals may be more competitive, assertive, and less concerned with the needs of others.

Neuroticism

This trait describes a person's tendency to experience negative emotions, such as anxiety, sadness, and worry [8]:

- **High neuroticism:** Individuals tend to be more emotionally reactive, anxious, and prone to negative emotions.
- **Low neuroticism:** Individuals tend to be more emotionally stable, calm, and resilient to stress.

The "easy child" may develop a personality high in openness, conscientiousness, extraversion, and agreeableness and low in neuroticism, while the "difficult" child may develop into the exact opposite. What's important to understand is that though a child may be born with an innate temperament, external forces, including caregivers, lived experiences, social support, and education, and internal forces, such as cognitive ability, shape personality throughout development. A child who may have been grouped in the "difficult" temperament category may develop high openness and extraversion due to a support system that encouraged continued exposure to new experiences.

Clinical Scenario A 12-year-old male presents to the emergency department after a fall resulting in an upper extremity fracture. He is very anxious and asking many questions about pain with a cast, need for surgery, if his arm will heal, time to healing, how sure the provider is that there is a fracture, etc. His parent is trying to tell him to "be quiet and let them do their job." In this situation, addressing the child directly, acknowledging their fears and anxiety and providing reassurance about the method for fixing the fracture, showing them the X-ray images, describing the healing process, and listening to them can make a big difference in comforting both the child and the anxious caregiver with them.

Personality Types

The philosopher Hippocrates proposed a theory to describe four temperaments associated with the four bodily "humors": sanguine, choleric, melancholic, and phlegmatic [9]. Modern theories have used the four-temperament theory to describe four personality types. Though separated into distinct categories, psychologists believe individuals share traits from a few if not all personality types.

Sanguine

The sanguine child tends to enjoy being sociable and outgoing. They seek creative outlets and spend time daydreaming. Emotionally, sanguine children can be described as sensitive and compassionate. They may lose attention on a task easily and may exhibit impulsive behaviors [9].

Core Traits of a Sanguine Child

Confident
Optimistic
Pleasant
Talkative
Extraverted
Influential

Creative
Impulsive
Distractible
Disorganized

Choleric

The choleric child is seen as a leader. They are goal oriented and passionate. Choleric children tend to have high energy and can display aggressive and domineering behaviors toward others. They may be inflexible and display lower levels of empathy [9].

Core Traits of a Choleric Child

Assertive
Passionate
Self-motivated
Energetic
Decisive
Goal oriented
Issues with control
Irritable
Impatient

Melancholic

The melancholic child is perceived as a deep thinker. They are considerate toward others and self-sacrificing. Melancholic children are highly creative. They prefer things to be organized and schedule oriented. They are prone to moodiness and have obsessive tendencies [9].

Core Traits of a Melancholic Child

Thoughtful
Organized
Analytical

Methodical
Loyal
Self-sacrificing
Creative
Obsessive
Pessimistic
Moody

Phlegmatic
The phlegmatic child has a relaxed demeanor. They are quiet and calm and can easily entertain themselves. Toward others, the phlegmatic child is accepting and affectionate. They are fearful of change and are prone to laziness, poor discipline, and displaying passive aggressiveness [9].

Core Traits of a Phlegmatic Child

Relaxed
Kind
Reliable
Observant
Affectionate
Unenthusiastic
Fearful of change
Not goal oriented

Conclusion

There are many factors that contribute to the development of a child's personality. Understanding the strengths and weaknesses of a child's personality type can help the provider and parents discover how best to encourage and support the child throughout their development. These personality types encompass both positive and negative characteristics which may become more pronounced in stressful situations. Furthermore, diagnoses such as

ADHD, autism, OCD, or other neuropsychiatric conditions can impact how these traits manifest. Recognizing these inherent differences can help guide communication strategies with the child and the caregiver so that the healthcare goals are able to be discussed and achieved.

Key Points

- Temperament describes a person's biologic predisposition to emotional display, motor activity, reactivity, and self-regulation patterns.
- Temperament contributes to a child personality, but as they move through various developmental stages, personality is influenced and developed by other external factors.
- A child may exhibit traits from multiple personality types and exhibit both positive and negative characteristics related to these.
- Recognition and understanding from the clinician allows for adjustment in the approach to the patient in order to promote good communication.

References

1. Thomas A, Chess S. Temperament and development. Brunner/Mazel; 1977.
2. Rothbart MK. Becoming who we are: temperament and personality in development. New York: Guilford; 2011.
3. Zentner M, Bates JE. Child temperament: an integrative review of concepts, research programs, and measures. Int J Dev Sci. 2008;2(1–2):7–3.
4. Vaziri Flais S. Caring for your school-age child: ages 5 to 12. 3rd ed. American Academy of Pediatrics; 2018.
5. Understanding your child's temperament: why it's important. HealthyChildren.org. 2009, November 2. https://www.healthychildren.org/English/ages-stages/gradeschool/Pages/How-to-Understand-Your-Childs-Temperament.aspx

6. Costa PT, McCrae RR. Age differences in personality structure: a cluster analytic approach. J Gerontol. 1976;
7. McCrae RR, John OP. An introduction to the five-factor model and its applications. J Pers. 1992;60(2):175–215.
8. Goldberg LR. The development of markers for the Big-five factor structure. Psychol Assess. 1992;4(1):26–42.
9. Merenda PF. Toward a four-factor theory of temperament and/or personality. J Pers Assess. 1987;51(3):367–74.

Unique Aspects of Care When the Patient Is Not the One Providing History or Implementing Care Plan

2

Somtochi Okafor

Introduction

The patient-physician relationship serves as the cornerstone of medicine that has built upon tenets of autonomy, beneficence, nonmaleficence, and justice. Patients entrust physicians with vulnerability and truth of their physical, mental, and emotional condition in hopes of alleviating their ailments. However, with pediatric care, this vulnerability and truth shape into a complex dynamic that requires multifaceted communication and advocacy. In general, these aspects of care are not merely relegated to pediatrics, but their nuanced manifestations within pediatrics remain unique in that the history, diagnosis, and treatment plan are primarily carried out and dependent on a third party who is not the patient. Thus, this chapter will delve into these unique aspects of care as well as offer considerations for discourse on improving the pediatric patient-physician relationship.

S. Okafor (✉)
Department of Head and Neck Surgery, Duke University School of Medicine, Durham, NC, USA
e-mail: Somtochi.Okafor@duke.edu

E. Raynor (ed.), *Managing Challenging Patients and Families in Health Care Settings*, https://doi.org/10.1007/978-3-032-10492-2_2

Multifaceted Communication

> Listen to your patient, [they are] telling you the diagnosis.
> Sir William Osler

Children remain one of the most vulnerable populations in our society. Thus, we as healthcare providers are nestled in a unique position to ensure and maintain patient advocacy, autonomy, and beneficence while understanding that the pediatric population may not have the legal or physical agency to advocate or communicate for themselves. As such, effective communication that reflects the patient, the parent,[1] caregiver, or guardian and the healthcare provider remains paramount. As Sir William Osler aptly stated, a patient's history is essential to the diagnosis and subsequent treatment of a patient. However, in the pediatric context, it is often the third party (i.e., parent, guardian, caretaker, etc.) who provides this to the healthcare provider. Several elements such as reliability, interpretation, and emotional transference must be considered when listening to the history as relayed by the third party. Brand and Dulemon conducted a systematic review on the reliability of obtaining a pediatric clinical history from parents and noted there were no studies found that investigated the reliability of parents' account of a patient's presentation [1]. The lack of such studies likely stems from the difficulty in developing a reference point or gold standard for a patient's personal experience, let alone a parent's perception of that [1]. Furthermore, this highlights the complexities of interpersonal subjectivity and the leveled tiers of communication that stem from not only the patient's subjective perception of their health but also that of their parent. How can providers interpret both the parents' telling of their child's experience while identifying and recognizing the child's physical presentation and subjective truth? Such a feat requires communication and mutual trust.

[1] For the sake of consistency and clarity, I will refer to pediatric patients' representative, parent, guardian, or caretaker as "parent," understanding the nuanced and complex relationship children may have with those who take them to healthcare provider appointments/evaluations.

Both parties, the healthcare provider and the parent, must maintain trust that the counterparty is working toward and/or representing the child's best interest. Various studies have investigated the nuances of patients' trust in healthcare providers and have identified communication as one of the main elements of developing trust in the patient-provider relationship [2–5]. This is multifaceted and not only includes verbal communication but also emphasizes the importance of nonverbal communication through body language and demeanor [4]. Consequently, the first impression a parent develops of the provider depends on the provider's ability to communicate their genuine intent to care for the patient, their clinical acumen, and overall their empathy toward the patient and their loved ones. Therefore, providers should recognize that the trajectory of the patient-physician relationship is initially dependent on the child's parents' confidence in the clinician.

Although the parents' trust in the provider forms the foundation of communication, healthcare providers must also develop a trust in the parents' telling of the clinical presentation. This trust relies upon the concordance of subjective perception and the realities of the child's clinical presentation. Researchers have investigated physicians' perception of patient's reliability in their clinical history, but these efforts have been limited to the adult world [2, 6]. Pelaccia et al. conducted a qualitative study that highlighted emergency room physicians' judgments of patient's reliability. This study revealed that physicians quickly "labeled" patients as either "reliable" or "unreliable" based on the consistency or inconsistency of their clinical history which ultimately resulted in a different course of action in eliciting a history [6]. These findings illustrate the impact physician judgment can impart on the patient-physician relationship. It is important to remember that provider bias whether conscious or unconscious can further impact this relationship. Providers should remain diligent in recognizing, identifying, and rectifying biases that may inhibit the delivery of equitable and appropriate care. Overall, when applying these considerations to pediatric patients, we must strive to maintain an open and considerate perception of parents' perspective while weighing them in alignment or contrast to the reality of a child's physical presentation.

Advocacy

> If we don't stand for children, then we don't stand for much.
> Marian Wright Edelman

In addition to appreciating the pivotal role that parents play in providing patient history, providers must also distinguish the critical importance of the mutual goal among both parents and providers: patient advocacy. Patient advocacy is the concept and practice of a third-party representative seeking to illuminate and address the concerns and interests of an individual or group who may not hold the same agency or power to speak for themselves. The advocate's role is to promote the "best interest" of the patient while representing the patient's desires as accurately as possible [7]. Thus, every parent who brings their child to clinic or surgery for medical evaluation and surgical intervention is by virtue an advocate for their child. Providers should consider that inherently the underlying premise of parents' clinical aim is to represent their child's ailment or concern to the best of their abilities while rectifying that their child may not be able to voice their own concerns.

While advocacy from the parental perspective predominantly involves traversing the barriers involved to bring the child to the clinic or hospital evaluation (i.e., missing work, spending money on gas or transportation fare, etc.) as well as vocalizing the issues affecting the child, physician advocacy pushes these experiences forward to involve developing and instituting a treatment plan as well as potentially lobbying for institutional or governmental change. One of the most prominent examples of this stems from Dr. Chevalier Jackson, one of the vital leaders and trailblazers in otolaryngology head and neck surgery. Throughout his decades-long career of developing and transforming endoscopy and bronchoscopy techniques to improve foreign body retrievals as well as treat caustic ingestion injury, Dr. Jackson advocated for federal legislation to codify required labeling for caustic substances after treating several hundred patients who accidentally ingested lye [8, 9]. Dr. Jackson was able to do so after spending nearly two decades documenting patient experiences, clinical progression, and prognosis after caustic ingestion as evidence to the federal government as examples of the dire need to label substances to prevent the deadly sequela of accidental ingestion [8]. Thus, his work illustrates the impact providers' advocacy can implement on a more powered scale.

Conclusion

Through dedicated and effective communication that is founded upon trust, both parents and providers can work together to form a coalition dedicated to treating pediatric patients. In doing so, both parties serve as advocates for children, who due to age, physical limitations, and minimal legal authority are not capable of doing so themselves. Inevitably, both groups fundamentally share the same vested interest and dedication to caring for and improving the well-being of children despite the initial differences.

Summary

- The patient-provider relationship in pediatrics is a complex dynamic that requires identification of the patient, patient's family or guardian, and the provider as cornerstones to facilitate communication.
- Multifaceted communication, advocacy, and understanding are unique aspects of care that both healthcare providers and parents must recognize and respect in efforts to care for pediatric patients.
- Both parents and providers must maintain a mutual level of trust to ensure and promote effective communication.
- Advocacy is paramount to pediatric care and very much defines its role in medicine. Both parents and providers must work together to promote patient advocacy as children do and may not have the legal or physical agency to advocate for themselves.

References

1. Brand PLP, van Dulmen S. Can we trust what parents tell us? A systematic review. Paediatr Respir Rev. 2017;24:65–71. https://doi.org/10.1016/j.prrv.2017.01.003.
2. Brennan N, Barnes R, Calnan M, Corrigan O, Dieppe P, Entwistle V. Trust in the health-care provider–patient relationship: a systematic mapping review of the evidence base. Int J Qual Health Care. 2013;25(6):682–8. https://doi.org/10.1093/intqhc/mzt063.
3. Dinç L, Gastmans C. Trust in nurse–patient relationships: a literature review. Nurs Ethics. 2013;20(5):501–16. https://doi.org/10.1177/0969733012468463.
4. Riva S, Monti M, Iannello P, Pravettoni G, Schulz PJ, Antonietti A. A preliminary mixed-method investigation of trust and hidden signals in medical consultations. PLoS One. 2014;9(3):e90941. https://doi.org/10.1371/journal.pone.0090941.
5. Street RL, O'Malley KJ, Cooper LA, Haidet P. Understanding concordance in patient-physician relationships: personal and ethnic dimensions of shared identity. Ann Fam Med. 2008;6(3):198–205. https://doi.org/10.1370/afm.821.
6. Pelaccia T, Tardif J, Triby E, et al. Do emergency physicians trust their patients? Intern Emerg Med. 2016;11(4):603–8. https://doi.org/10.1007/s11739-016-1410-1.
7. Brazg T, Lindhorst T, Dudzinski D, Wilfond B. Defining patient advocacy for the context of clinical ethics consultation: a review of the literature and recommendations for consultants. J Clin Ethics. 2016;27(2):176–84. https://doi.org/10.1086/jce2016272176.
8. Eriksson SE, Jobe BA, Ayazi S. Chevalier Jackson: father of endoscopic surgery, and champion of women in medicine, social justice, and public health. Surg Endosc. 2023;37(9):6660–71. https://doi.org/10.1007/s00464-023-10256-x.
9. Tucker JA, Reilly BK, Tucker ST, Reilly JS. Pediatric otolaryngology in the United States: Chevalier Jackson's legacy for the 21st century. Otolaryngol Head Neck Surg. 2012;146(1):5–7. https://doi.org/10.1177/0194599811426678.

3 Who Decides? Navigating Medical Decision-Making and Caregiver Challenges for Minors and Adults Needing Assistance

Shelia Rittgers

Medical Decision-Making for Children Whose Caregiver Is Not the Parent

Background

In the United States, there are an estimated 3.7 million children living in a home without a parent as their primary caregiver [1]. Most are with family members with the large number being grandparents. It is estimated that between the years of 2005 and 2015, 2.9 million children were being cared for by their grandparents [2]. Other children may be cared for by relatives such as aunts and uncles or by close friends of the parents.

In caring for a child, providing shelter, food, and a safe environment does not automatically equate to being able to legally seek and consent for healthcare or even enroll a child in school. Practitioners are legitimately concerned about liability when someone who is not a biological parent is making decisions for a

S. Rittgers (✉)
Duke University Health System, Durham, NC, USA

E. Raynor (ed.), *Managing Challenging Patients and Families in Health Care Settings*, https://doi.org/10.1007/978-3-032-10492-2_3

child. Not being able to participate in medical care is a challenge for families and other caregivers. Many must then find other means to obtain the authority they need to make medical decisions for a minor. This can be done by completing a power of attorney document that outlines the responsibilities another adult will be taking on for the minor such as healthcare and/or education, or an individual can become the legally appointed guardian or custodian through the court system. Some states offer legislative options such as the North Carolina Statute Authorization to Consent to Healthcare for a Minor (N.C G.S. 32A-34) that can be completed and allows the individual caring for the minor to consent to medical treatment. The North Carolina Consent Statute [3] and the power of attorney documents need the signature of the custodial parent and must be notarized to be recognized as legally valid. Some states have enacted consenting laws after noting that relatives or friends have great difficulty not only seeking educational and medical treatment for children in their care but also maintaining positive relationships with the parents. Consenting laws allow the person caring for the child to complete an affidavit under oath stating that they are the primary caregiver for the child, thus avoiding going to court for guardianship or completing a power of attorney or state consent statute that has to be signed by the parent. Although these affidavits do not give the caregiver legal custody or guardianship of a child, they do allow the caregiver to enroll a child in school and seek medical treatment. These documents need to be notarized but do not require a parent's signature. The affidavits can be rescinded by parents. There is a penalty of perjury if the information provided by the caregiver is false. Some states only allow relatives to complete these affidavits, while others will accept the affidavit of a nonrelative. The American Bar Association provides detailed information on states consenting laws [4]. Neither the affidavit, the power of attorney, nor the legislative consenting document gives guardianship of the minor child to another person, but they do allow another individual to seek medical care for that child within the guidelines of what is written in the document by the custodial parent.

Appointing a Legal Guardian/Custodian for a Minor

The appointment of a guardian or legal custodian is an action of the court that takes considerable time. A petition is filed (usually in the county where the child resides) and a hearing set where a judge hears evidence as to why a child's parents should no longer have custody of the child. If the judge agrees, someone other than the parent is appointed to be responsible for caring for and making decisions for the child. The person seeking guardianship of a child is often a relative or a close friend. This person is called the legal guardian although some states refer to the person as the conservator or even legal custodian. This varies from state to state. The responsibilities given to the person appointed as guardian are the most important aspect of the court order. These responsibilities may be broad or limited and often include authorizing and consenting to healthcare, enrollment in school, meeting other basic needs, day-to-day care, and finances. The responsibilities depend on what type of guardian was appointed—for example, guardian of the person or guardian of the estate—and the language used in the order. The court order will determine the extent of the involvement of the guardian in the healthcare of the child. It is wise to see if the guardianship is temporary or permanent as there may be a need to return to court for final disposition and to make sure that one has the most current court order. In most cases, parental rights are not terminated when a legal guardian/custodian is appointed as that is a separate court action. It is simply that the appointed guardian/custodian is given authority to make decisions for the child. Again what is explicitly written in the order with respect to healthcare decision-making is what needs to be looked at closely. Although developed to assist refugee families caring for a non-biological child, the Bridging Refugee Youth and Children's Services (BRYCS) has information on the guardianship process for all states [5].

In summary, other options exist beyond legal guardianship or custody including power of attorney, consenting affidavits, and state healthcare consenting statutes.

Case Scenario I

A 10-year-old Jesse is brought to a clinic visit by his grandmother. She states that she is his guardian and has been caring for him for 7 years. She adds that his aunts and an uncle also care for him. Although it is not urgent, he will need a tonsillectomy and adenoidectomy. You need consent. You note in the electronic medical record that he is followed by a primary care practice in your health system. The grandmother as well as an aunt and one uncle have been bringing him to those appointments and engaging with staff about his care, but you cannot find a legal court document in the record noting that the grandmother or any other relative has legal custody/guardianship of Jesse. You ask the grandmother for this document, and she reminds you that she has been caring for him for 7 years as his mother is "in and out of the picture" and she does not know where his father is and no one has ever asked her about this. She comments that in her culture, family members assume care for children if their parents are unable to care for them and make decisions about all their needs. Eventually she states that she does not have any formal paperwork. In the grandmother's mind, she is Jesse's guardian. **What do you do?**

Case Scenario II

Paulie is a 4-year-old female with a history of hearing loss. She will need a sedated evaluation. You receive a call from pre-op staff with questions about information they gathered from the caregivers who identify themselves as the adoptive parents. There is concern that the caregivers are not the adoptive parents as the medical and social history they share is confusing. The presumed adoptive parents provide a paper that states that the biological parents have given the patient to the caregivers to be adopted by them. The letter is signed and dated at the time that the patient would have been 1 year of age**. What do you do?**

In looking at the first scenario, it is important to understand the family culture and dynamics and how this impacts the caregiver's understanding of what it means to have the authority to legally make medical decisions for a child. You need to know who the legal medical decision-maker for a child is when the child is not living with their parent even if the caregiver is a relative. Depending on what state you are in, there may be several options to obtain consent. If mom is available by phone, witnessed consent can be obtained. In all states, one can ask the grandmother to speak to the mother about completing a power of attorney (POA) focusing on healthcare decisions. These are often referred to as medical or healthcare power of attorney documents. Many clear and concise forms can be found online, or one can seek out an attorney for advice. In a state such as North Carolina, there is state legislation to assist with this type of situation. It is called the authorization to consent to healthcare of a minor statute, and the parent can complete the form and provide it to medical staff. In Jesse's situation, the mother can complete and sign either of these documents, and the grandmother will be able to participate in and consent to care. These forms must be notarized. If you are in a state that allows a consenting affidavit, where the grandmother can swear that she is the primary caregiver for the child, this can also be done. The mother does not have to sign this, but it must be notarized. If the mother cannot be reached and is not readily available for this appointment or other needs for the patient, Jesse's grandmother could petition the court for guardianship/custody as this would legally place the patient in her care and the mother would have to return to court to change the decision. It solidifies the place of the grandmother in caring for and making decisions for the child without worry that the mother would suddenly take the child from the grandmother's home. If the medical care is seen as urgent, most states have a relative consent hierarchy that can be followed. However, this does not solve the issue of who has legal guardianship or consent authorization in the future. Regardless of what document they choose to use (POA, state consenting statute, or consenting affidavit), you need to obtain a copy of it, place it in the record, make note of who has authorization to consent, and proceed with getting consent from the legally responsible person.

The second scenario brings to one's attention that some individuals who are caring for a child may call themselves the "adoptive parent" or even a relative such as a "grandparent" but they are neither. It is wise to get clarification on this matter. In Paulie's situation, the parents thought that if they wrote a letter dictating what they wanted to do with respect to Paulie's care and upbringing and had the paper notarized, that was all that was required of them. They did not go through a legal adoption nor any other process (power of attorney/consenting affidavit/state consenting statute) to give the caregivers the authority to seek and make medical decisions on behalf of the child. You may be given a paper stating that the biological parent of the patient has given guardianship to or has given up their rights to the current caregiver so the child can be "adopted," but that does not make it legal. Both of these processes are legal actions and must be heard in court. One cannot simply give one's child to another person without the safety, care, and well-being of that child being assessed in the court. When adoptions are finalized, the family will receive an adoption decree. If the practice does not receive any legal paperwork, one will need to provide the current caregiver information on the different options that will allow them to give authorization for medical treatment and/or seek legal guardianship. Alternatively, your practice can reach out to the parent if they are available for witnessed consent by phone and also provide the parent with options that would allow the child's current caregiver to seek and consent to treatment of the patient.

Although not rising to the same level as consenting to care, seeking medical care can also be a challenge when done in the absence of a parent or guardian. It is not uncommon especially in primary care for a relative or friend to bring a child to an appointment if the parent is unable to do it. Health institutions should have a policy that both abides by HIPAA standards and also makes every effort to allow the institution to provide care to the minor. A common protocol is to have the parent write a letter stating that they cannot attend the appointment, naming who is with the child and stating that the institution has permission to see the child and treat, and share protected health information with the responsible adult who has brought the child to the clinic. The parent should sign the letter and provide a contact number in case they need to be reached to discuss additional treatments. Phone verification is another means to obtain permission to see and treat a minor who is not with their parent. The call is made by two clinical staff and documented. If it appears that a more permanent plan is needed, the staff could speak to the parent and caregiver about completing a power of attorney document, a state healthcare consenting statute, or a consenting affidavit. It is important to know the policy of the healthcare institution and the laws of the state in which one practices that pertain to seeking and treating a minor in the absence of the parent or court-appointed legally responsible adult.

Parental Custody and Medical Decision-Making

Background

Parents are considered a child's custodians because they are biological relatives of the child. Custody is often a term used for outlining responsibility and decision-making for a child whose parents are either divorced or not together but have paternity established, as both have parental rights. There are different types of custody as outlined below by the Cornell Law School's Legal Information Institute:

> A custodial parent is the parent that lives with and cares for their minor child for all (sole physical custody) or most (primary physical custody) of the time. This contrasts with the noncustodial parent, who might have the child on a limited basis or only have visitation rights. Some parents split physical custody equally in a joint custody arrangement, in which case both would be considered custodial parents. This type of arrangement can be made informally by the agreement of both parents or through the courts in a custody lawsuit. Physical custody differs from legal custody, which is the right to make important decisions for and about the child. Custodial parents who have sole physical custody and sole legal custody are deemed to have sole custody and need not consult the noncustodial parent in decision-making. A custodial parent might instead share legal custody with the noncustodial parent; called joint legal custody, this means the parents must consult each other on major issues about the child regardless of who the child lives with. In either case, custodial parents are often required to follow court orders regarding the noncustodial parent, such as facilitating visitation or not moving out of a certain location without approval [6].

Addressing Disagreements with Recommended Care

As noted above, if both parents have joint legal custody, the court order (also known as custody agreement) can provide information on medical decision-making and what is to be done if parents cannot come to a mutual decision about healthcare needs. It is expected that parents will work together, but that is not always the case. If the parents are struggling to come to an agreement about treatment, it is imperative for the provider to continue to communicate with both parents, addressing any barriers that are preventing the care needed, and try to resolve the issue.

If the conflict between the parents about the recommended care cannot be reconciled, it becomes important to have a copy of the custody agreement in order to see what kind of decision authority has been given to the parents. Some parents may extend themselves more authority than they have been given in the custody document. During a dispute over care, reviewing a copy of the custody order will allow one to see if the parents must come to a mutual agreement on medical care or if there is a statement in the order giving one parent the final decision-making authority for medical needs. The language used in the court order will dictate next steps with respect to moving forward with treatment for the child. If one parent is not given the final decision-making authority for medical care in the custody order, the parent that wishes to proceed with treatment may need to return to court and request that amendments to the order be heard.

Case Scenario I

Willie is a 6-year-old male with a history of Chiari malformation and will need surgery. His parents are divorced. His mother states that she has sole legal custody of Willie and wants no information shared with his father. Two days after the clinic visit, his father calls the office asking for a review of the clinic visit. The nursing and office staff tell the father that they cannot share health information with him as they are basing this on the information they received from the mother. He is angry and upset stating that he has rights and wants to know about his son's health issues. **What do you do?**

It is important to obtain a copy of the parental custody order agreement so it can be reviewed. Your practice can call Willie's mother to request the custody order so the practice can follow it. The practice can also call Willie's father to request the custody order. Upon review, the custody order states that the mother has sole legal and physical custody of Willie, and the father has visitation access. However, there is nothing in the order that states that medical information cannot be shared with the father nor have his parental rights been terminated. With his rights intact and nothing written in the order stating that medical information cannot be shared, the father can be given his son's health information. The mother as sole custodian has the authority to make medical decisions for Willie, but the mother cannot prevent health information from being shared with the father. There is nothing in the custody order stating that this cannot be done and the father still has his parental rights. What is written in a custody order will guide how one responds to a situation. It is good to remember that all states have similar statutes that dictate terms of custody law. Custody law statutes are careful to make sure that a parent has access to their child's medical and educational information, unless it is otherwise ordered.

Total Medical Compliance has a brief review of health information and custody issues that provides details on releasing medical information [7].

Case Scenario II

Gina is a 9-year-old with asthma. Her parents are not married. They have been through court to establish a custody agreement. Paternity has been established. The custody agreement states that both parents have joint legal and physical custody of her. Because they have joint legal custody, they are to make major decisions such as educational, general welfare, dental, and nonemergency medical decisions together. There have been issues with the parents disagreeing on her treatment plan. The father wishes to proceed with recommended care, but the mother does not. Several attempts to answer questions and provide information on the need for treatment have not brought about any resolution and the standoff is beginning to impact her health. **What do you do?**

As with the first scenario, it will be important to ask for a copy of the court custody agreement. Upon review of the agreement, it is written that if the parents cannot reach a decision with respect to healthcare needs, the defendant—in this case the father—has the final decision-making authority. In circumstances like this, having the court order is imperative to help discern how to move forward when there is an impasse regarding medical care.

Parental custody disputes can make providing care difficult and sometimes exasperating. It is a delicate balance between listening and acknowledging the struggles between the parents and remaining a neutral observer. The focus remains on the needs of the most important person in the room: the child. Encourage the parents to leave their personal hostilities aside as you, the provider, point out not only the medical needs but also the emotional needs of the child during a time that may be anxiety provoking for them. You may also want to reach out to your institutional risk management group as needed, and if you have access to a clinical social worker, partner with them on how to engage the parents, understand court orders, and manage what can be a very stressful situation.

Custody with the Department of Social Services (Foster Care and Relative Caregivers) and Medical Decision-Making

Background

Although the numbers are consistently decreasing, the number of children in foster care in the United States at the end of FY 2022 was 368,500, compared to 392,000 children in foster care at the end of FY 2021 [8]. Children in foster care are exposed to early trauma that can include witnessing domestic violence or being victims of abuse and/or neglect. In July 2021, the American Academy of Pediatrics issued a statement on children in foster care estimating that about 50% have chronic physical problems (e.g., asthma, anemia, visual loss, hearing loss, and neurological disorders), approximately 10% are medically fragile or complex, and many have a history of prenatal (maternal) substance exposure and/or premature birth [9]. This has led to the American Academy of Pediatrics to recognize foster children as a special patient group.

There are very clear standards on the situations in which Departments of Social Services (also known as DSS, Department of Human Services, or Child Welfare Departments) can take custody of children and remove them from their homes: high risk of abuse, immediate threat of harm, and neglect. The department must file a petition with the court system that provides evidence of maltreatment and supports the fact that the child is not safe in the home. A judge will decide if the department has provided evidence in the petition that demonstrates that the child is at substantial risk of harm or has been harmed or has been neglected or is dependent and can no longer remain in the home as it is a safety risk. In this case, the department is given legal custody of the child by means of an order for custody. Then the department starts a broader investigation into the reasons that led to the removal and works with a family to address these concerns with the first option being a plan to return the child to the home.

When a child is removed from the home, DSS usually attempts to locate a family member who can provide safe care; if this is not possible, the child is placed in foster care. In general foster caregivers or family members (often called kinship caregivers) can seek routine care for a patient and emergency care if needed as this is what is often dictated through state laws when a child is in the custody of the Department of Social Services and placed into care. Once a child is placed, a foster family or kinship family will be provided a verification of custody letter that explains who has custody of the child and who to contact about any treatment needs. Even though these caregivers can seek routine/emergency care, they cannot sign for treatments such as psychotropic medication, psychological care, some immunizations, or procedures that require informed consent because they are not the legal guardian. It is not uncommon for those providing kinship care or foster care to be confused by this limited decision-making as they see themselves as the child's custodian, and although the child is in their physical custody, they do not have legal custody or guardianship which would give them the authority to consent to treatment.

If consent for treatment is needed, there are different means to obtaining authorization for the children in the custody of social services, most of which are driven by court decree or the laws of the state in which the child lives. One action is for the director of DSS or their designee to complete consents for a child (oral or written). When this occurs, it is usually due to a parent giving the director permission to consent to care that is outside of what is seen as routine or seeking emergency care, or there is a court order authorizing this. Other departments will cosign consents with the child's parents, and there are also those who will not sign any consents but will request that a parent be contacted and informed of the medical need and complete any consents. It is important to work with the social worker from the social services department to understand their policies and the state custody laws when it comes to getting consent for a child in their custody, as the court ruling for removal can provide initial information on who can consent for the child's care and treatment and what kind of care can be authorized.

Case Scenario

Faith is a 6-year-old with an autoimmune disease. She is in the custody of the county Department of Social Services. They are working with the parent on reunification. She has been with her foster caregiver for 10 months. The medication prescribed needs to be changed as it is no longer effective in treating her disease. The provider and clinic social worker have informed the social services department social worker that a new medication needs to be started and why this is necessary. The social services social worker has spoken to the mother about the needed change. The mother refuses to consent to the new medication. The provider has given information to the mother about why a new medication is needed trying to address all parental concerns. Two months pass and the parent continues to refuse to consent to the new medication. This is impacting Faith's well-being. She continues to show increased disease activity that is impacting her function and her emotional health. Due to the impact on Faith's health, the DSS department director, who is open to starting a new treatment, has stated that the agency will pursue a court order to obtain permission for the new medication, as it is in the best interest of the child. **What do you do?**

When a child in custody of the Department of Social Services is first seen by your practice, it is important to obtain a copy of the custody certification and to gather contact information for the social worker assigned to the child's case. This will allow you to not only work with the foster parent or family member who is caring for the child but also keep the social worker assigned to the family up to date on the child's treatment and any needed changes and answer any questions about the child's care as they are the legal custodians of the child. In Faith's case, detailed chart documentation will need to show that the current medication regimen is no longer effective and new medication is recommended, noting the medical and any emotional impact to the child. Due diligence needs to be made to try to engage the parent in the child's care. If this has failed, talk with the DSS social worker about the agency returning to court to obtain an order to start the new medication. All of this should be documented. The DSS social worker will request clinic notes and possibly a letter from the provider explaining the disease process and why a new medication is needed. This will be submitted to the court by DSS as they will request an order giving them authorization to approve the medication change. The judge in these circumstances is looking at what is best for the child and with proper documentation will often honor the request. With the court's approval, the provider can begin the new medication regimen.

Working with social services can be complex. Not only are they charged with ensuring care and safety for a child, they are also working with the family on reunification. This may impact who signs consents and makes decisions about care. Good communication with the DSS social worker is vital for several reasons: first, to know who can consent to care; second, to know the family reunification plan; and, third, to have assistance with engaging the parent in care prior to a child returning home. Collaborating with the DSS social worker allows you the opportunity to engage the parent in the child's treatment, discuss the child's diagnosis, and address any questions the parent may have, so the parent can be ready to assume the role of caregiver and follow the treatment plan when the child returns to their home.

Addressing Medical Decision-Making for Young Adults with Intellectual and Developmental Disabilities: Guardianship and Other Support Options

Background

Parents are the custodians of their children who are minors. Parents and others may believe that they are automatically the guardian of their young adult child with an intellectual and developmental disability when they turn 18 but they are not. When a child turns 18, they are recognized as a legal adult. It is presumed that the individual is responsible for their own decisions and parents are no longer considered the medical decision-makers. Decisions about healthcare are then made between a provider and the young adult with a parent being included only at the request of the young adult.

For the young adult with an intellectual and developmental disability and concern for capacity, there is a legal process that will determine if they need to have a guardian appointed (some states use the word conservator). The guardianship process for adults is described in greater detail below. The court system will determine if the young adult is competent to safely manage their own affairs. If found incompetent, the court will appoint a guardian. The court determines who will be appointed as a general guardian (over the person and estate) or guardian of the estate (manages business and finances of person) or guardian of the person (focuses on issues related to the care and custody of the young adult), which is the most common appointment. The person to whom a guardian is appointed is often referred to as the "ward." The appointed guardian is now responsible to care for and mak decisions (healthcare, basic needs, legal, living arrangements) that are in the best interest of the ward. They are also tasked with allowing the ward to continue to participate in decision-making as much as is within their comprehension. Over 1.3 million people in the United States have a legal guardian [10]. There are options other than full guardianship of an individual; this is referred to as limited guardianship. While the majority of guardians appointed by the court are family members, there are also state guardians and private guardians.

There is serious impact to a person's civil rights when they are appointed a guardian. In seven states, adults who have been appointed a legal guardian cannot vote, while in other states these individuals cannot drive or get married [11]. Over the last decade, disability rights advocates as well as congressional representatives such as Senators Elizabeth Warren and Bob Casey, Jr., have been advocating for more oversight for the guardianship process as well as more decision-making options for individuals who with additional support can retain some autonomy and their civil rights [12].

Guardianship law varies across the states. Guardianship is pursed when there are no other options that could better protect the rights of an individual when capacity is a concern. The United States Department of Justice provides information on state law and the guardianship process [13]. The *Journal of Financial Service Professionals* (Vol. 75, No. 1 (2012) | pp. 59–79) also provides a review of the guardianship laws of all 50 states.

Guardianship Process for Adults

The guardianship process starts when a petition is filed in court stating that an individual cannot care for themselves, they are unable to make decisions, or their ability to make decisions is so limited that it puts them at risk of harm; therefore, they require a guardian. In many states, this is most often done through the Clerk of Superior Court. Petitions are usually filed by family members or professionals such as social workers from social services agencies if the young adult in need has no relative to care for them. The court system refers to the person (or people) filing the petition as the "petitioner(s)" and the person alleged to be incompetent as the "respondent." There is due process, and in some states a guardian ad litem is appointed to meet with the respondent. It is their role to advocate in the best interest of the person. Not all states require an attorney, but it is recommended if the respondent is contesting the petition. A hearing is set, and the Clerk of Superior Court may ask for supportive documentation to review prior to the hearing. The respondent will be served by the local sheriff's office as it is required that they are informed that they are involved in a legal action. At the hearing, there must be clear and convincing evidence submitted supporting the petition that the respondent is not capable of caring for themselves. The respondent's physician can submit an affidavit or a letter that speaks to the capacity of the individual. This is not a requirement of all states, but it is important to know the laws for guardianship of the state in which one practices. The Clerk of Court usually makes their decision at the end of the hearing. This process depending on the state where the person is residing can take up to 30 days. There are options for filing an interim guardianship if the Clerk of Court can be given information that supports the urgency of the situation. A hearing will then be held as soon as possible.

Many states offer what is called limited guardianship. It is an option for those individuals who do not need the broad oversight of full guardianship. The individual may need assistance with complex decisions such as medical or financial decisions but can manage other needs. Limited guardianship focuses on the abilities and the needs of the individual. The court order for limited guardianship is written with those needs in mind. This process is completed through the court system like full guardianship and may be an option suggested by a guardian ad litem or the petitioner.

Supported decision-making (SDM) is an alternative to guardianship that more states are implementing in order to provide the least restrictive impact on an individual's right to self-determination. In supported decision-making, an individual with a disability but with presumed capacity can talk with someone they trust about their needs. The individual can receive assistance in decision-making with respect to their healthcare, finances, and personal affairs. The individual can discuss how they best learn and the kind of help they need. The purpose is to support the individual to be able to make their own decisions. An agreement can then be written up naming those whom the individual trusts to help them, the areas where assistance is needed, and how disagreements between the person and the trusted advocates will be managed. Many states have passed legislation to provide a legal path for supported decision-making as an alternative to guardianship and provide examples for the creation of this document [14].

The following table (Table 3.1) highlights different decision-making options for the state of North Carolina [15]. Most states have similar options. Presumed capacity is the guideline for supportive decision-making, healthcare power of attorney, and advanced directives. Being named a representative payee (done through the social security administration) is not the same as being appointed a legal guardian.

Appointed guardians of young adults sometimes assume that guardianship of their young adult child would transfer to another state if they were to move. This is not correct. There is a process guardians must follow to transfer guardianship due to differences in state laws.

To reduce the complications that can come from moving to another state, the UAGPPJA (Uniform Adult Guardianship and Protective Proceedings Jurisdiction Act) was created to standardize the process of transferring guardianship form one state to another. Presently passed by 37 states, Puerto Rico, and the District of Columbia, the UAGPPJA streamlines the transfer process by stipulating that the substantive findings of the originating state be recognized and adopted by the new jurisdiction [16]. It is usually best for a family to obtain an attorney to assist with this transfer process and to provide guidance if there is no reciprocity between the state where the person was found incompetent and the state where the person is now living.

Table 3.1 Examples of decision-making options

Supported decision-making	Can be a formal or informal agreement. Would notarize if the agreement is formal	Person involved in their own decision-making and receives support when needed	Person and their advisors determine and document when support is needed
Advanced directives	Person makes their own decisions	Document states medical-mental health choices of the person for others to make if they are incapacitated	It is a legal document. Can be completed with an attorney, but this is not required
Representative payee	Formal process of appointment by agencies such as social security for those receiving benefits	Person receives support from another individual to manage state and federal benefits	Outside of government financial benefit, the person makes decisions for themselves. This is not legal guardianship
Power of attorney	Person participates in decision-making	Person states who will make decisions for them as defined in the document	It is a legal document. Often prepared with the assistance of an attorney
Guardianship	Person's ability to make decisions for themselves is limited	A petition is filed in court, and a hearing will determine if the individual is incapacitated	The court will determine the need for a guardian and the type of guardian and legally appoint a guardian

Case Scenario

Daryl is a 21-year-old male with a history of global developmental delay and seizures. He is nonverbal and requires total care. He is nonambulatory. He is being evaluated for surgery. He is brought to the clinic by his parents. Because of his age, and presentation, the staff ask about guardianship documents. The parents remind the staff that they are his parents and have cared for him all his life. They do not have any paperwork and ask what guardianship is. **What do you do?**

In this situation, it will be important for the parents to understand that although they will always be Daryl's parents, legally Daryl is considered an adult, and they can no longer make decisions for him. Explain the process of seeking adult guardianship and how it is used to assure that Daryl will have people caring for him for the duration of his life. If guardianship is granted to Daryl's parents, this will allow them to continue to make medical decisions for him. The family will need to obtain and complete a guardianship petition from the Clerk of Courts in the county in which they reside, or they can hire an attorney to assist them. Once the court decision on guardianship is made, ask the parents to bring the court order to the practice where Daryl receives care so it can be filed and documentation can be completed stating that Daryl's parents are his guardians.

As a provider, it is better to be proactive than reactive in situations where a guardian or some form of healthcare decision-making option is going to be needed for a young adult with an intellectual developmental disability or another disability that impacts capacity. If guardianship is clearly warranted, some states, such as North Carolina, allow the petition for guardianship to be initiated at age 17 and a half. It will be heard and a decision made by the court that will go into effect on the person's 18th birthday [17]. Some states now have an online process for starting this petition so needed forms can be completed online instead of going to the local courthouse to obtain them.

All children's care needs change as they grow older. Children with intellectual and developmental disabilities especially need someone advocating for their best interests as they age since they may not be able to advocate for themselves. Practitioners must speak to families about anticipated future care for special needs children as those children become young adults. For some families, the legal guardianship process will best meet the child's needs. For others, a form of decision-making assistance such as the Healthcare Power of Attorney or SDM is best.

Guidelines for Your Practice

In our society, it is becoming more common for people other than parents to be seeking medical care for minors in their care. Non-parental caregivers sometimes believe that they can make medical decisions for the child in their care. This kind of benevolent network can provide a broader support system for the family but it can also bring forth challenges for a provider. These are caregivers whether related to the patient or not who have taken on the immediate daily care of a child who also feel responsible for health related needs. Similarly, both parents and non-parental caregivers of young adults with intellectual disabilities feel responsible for medical decisions for this adult who is in their care. There are some cultures where caregivers have a shared responsibility to be involved in making treatment decisions for children in their care, so this may need to be taken into consideration when meeting a patient whose caregiver is not their parent but in their culture is expected to make all decisions related to the needs of the child. Below are some key points to remember when meeting a child who is accompanied to an appointment by someone other than a parent, when discussing who can make medical decisions, and when an adult with capacity issues is being seen by your practice:

1. **Clarifying roles and responsibilities.** Identify who is with the child, who is the primary medical decision-maker, and who has legal authority to make those decisions. Obtain the paperwork that explains who can make medical decisions for the child and document it. It is equally important to know who can legally make decisions for an adult with capacity concerns regardless of whether they are with a parent or another caregiver, as an adult with significant capacity issues needs to have a legal guardian appointed for them.
2. **Know your institution's policies and your state's laws on medical decision-making.** Be prepared to communicate the institution's policies and the laws associated with protected health information and medical decision-making or consenting. You will need to get a release of information from a parent

in order to share protected information with a relative or friend who will be involved in the patient's care but isn't the primary or legal decision-maker. Call a parent to get permission to see and treat a minor who comes for an appointment with someone other than the parent.

3. **Explain all options**. You may need to provide information on state consenting statutes, power of attorney forms, legal guardianship, or consenting affidavits if a parent wants a non-parental caregiver to be involved in making medical decisions and consenting to treatment for their child. Explaining these options will help the child's caregiver and parent decide what option works best for their situation.
4. **Talk to families with special needs teen about future care.** For teens with capacity concerns approaching the age of 16, engage in a conversation with the family and the teen if appropriate about what it means to be recognized as a legal adult and how that impacts medical decision-making. For those who do not have clear global capacity concerns, options such as a supported decision-making document can keep the patient engaged in their care. A healthcare power of attorney document can help the patient and family decide who can make medical decisions for the patient if the patient becomes unable to communicate their wishes. For those with serious global impairments and who will need some type of legal guardianship, the family can begin to prepare for that court process.

Addressing custody, guardianship, and caregiver concerns when establishing care with a patient is an important step in ensuring that you and the family or caregiver are on the same page regarding who has legal decision-making authority for a child or young adult with decision-making capacity concerns. There are several options outlined in this chapter that will allow a parent to give another person the authority to make medical decisions for their child and give guidance when facing situations where parents who share custody are not in agreement with treatment. There are options to assist parents and caregivers of young adults with capacity issues to prepare for future care and oversight of medical decisions.

Building a relationship with your risk management office and working with a clinic social worker if one is available can be very helpful. Their knowledge of guardianship and custody laws and other supported decision-making and consenting options can provide you support with these challenging situations.

Ensuring clarity on who can consent to a patient's treatment allows you to continue to put the patient first. You play a crucial role in helping families access the documentation they need in order to have others involved in medical decision-making and maintain integrity and accountability for all involved in the patient's care.

References

1. The Annie E. Casey Foundation, KIDS COUNT Data Center: Children Living With Neither Parent in the United States, 20172021. Accessed 1 June 2023. https://datacenter.aecf.org/data/tables/111-children-living-with-neither-parent#detailed/1/any/false/2048,1729,37,871,870,573,869,36,868,867/any/439,440
2. The Annie E. Casey Foundation, KIDS COUNT Data Center: Children in the Care of Grandparents in United States. Accessed 26 June 2023. https://datacenter.aecf.org/data/tables/108-children-in-the-care-of-grandparents?loc=1&loct=2#detailed/1/any/false/573,869,36,868,867,133,17,16/any/433,434.
3. North Carolina General Legislation. https://www.ncleg.net/EnactedLegislation/Statutes/PDF/ByArticle/Chapter_32A/Article_4.pdf
4. American Bar Association. https://www.americanbar.org/groups/public_interest/child_law/resources/child_law_practiceonline/child_law_practice/vol-33/june-2014/state-educational-and-health-care-consent-laws/
5. Bridging Refugee Youth and Children's Services. https://brycs.org/guardianship-information-by-state/
6. Legal Information Institute. https://www.law.cornell.edu/wex/custodial_parent
7. Total Medical Compliance. https://totalmedicalcompliance.com/minors-medical-records/
8. US Government Administration for Children and Families. https://www.acf.hhs.gov/media/press/2024/new-data-shows-consistent-decrease-children-foster-care
9. American Academy of Pediatrics. https://www.aap.org/en/patient-care/foster-care/physical-health-needs-of-children-in-foster-care/

10. Rethinking Guardianship To Protect Disabled People's Reproductive Rights. https://www.americanprogress.org/article/rethinking-guardianship-to-protect-disabled-peoples-reproductive-rights/
11. Ibid.
12. Warren E, Warren Jr BC. Casey Urge HHS, DOJ to provide more data on conservatorships and guardianships authorized by States. 1 Jul 2021. Available at https://www.warren.senate.gov/oversight/letters/warren-casey-urge-hhs-doj-to-provide-more-data-on-conservatorships-and-guardianships-authorized-by-states.
13. United States Department of Justice. https://www.justice.gov/elderjustice/guardianship-key-concepts-and-resources#appointed
14. National Resource Center for Supported Decision Making. https://supporteddecisionmaking.org/
15. North Carolina Department of Health and Human Services. https://www.ncdhhs.gov/decision-making-support-options
16. Special Needs Alliance. https://www.specialneedsalliance.org/blog/transferring-guardianship-between-states/
17. North Carolina Judicial Branch. https://www.nccourts.gov/help-topics/guardianship/guardianship

Impact of Health Literacy on Physician-Patient and Family Communication

4

Eileen Raynor

Definition of Health Literacy

Health literacy (HL) is difficult to fully define as it involves multiple factors that cross between overall literacy, numeric literacy, critical thinking skills, and overall motivation. Engagement with the healthcare system and familiarity with health and disease also factor into overall HL. Several definitions have been described in the literature.

Weiss describes HL as the "degree to which individuals have the capacity to obtain, process, and understand basic health information and services needed to make appropriate health decisions. It involves the ability to use and interpret text, documents, and numbers effectively." These are skills that might seem to be distinct but are highly correlated with one another [2]. According to Nutbeam [3], HL comprises three levels: basic or functional HL such as sufficient reading and writing skills, interactive HL that is the ability to extract health-relevant information and comprehend different communication methods, and, finally, critical HL that is

E. Raynor (✉)
Head and Neck Surgery & Communication Sciences, Duke University Health, Durham, NC, USA
e-mail: eileen.raynor@duke.edu

E. Raynor (ed.), *Managing Challenging Patients and Families in Health Care Settings*, https://doi.org/10.1007/978-3-032-10492-2_4

described as the more advanced skills needed to critically analyze health-relevant information and to use it for healthcare decision-making [3, 4].

Health literacy is "linked to literacy and entails people's knowledge, motivation and competences to access, understand, appraise, and apply health information in order to make judgments and take decisions in everyday life concerning healthcare, disease prevention and health promotion to maintain or improve quality of life during the life course." Moreover, an individual's HL depends upon their personal situation including their health status, risks, or problems, their affiliation with social group(s) (e.g., health practitioners, patients, and different age groups), and other socioeconomic determinants [5]. A systematic review by Von Boxel found 12 different definitions for HL with some specific focuses. It evolves over time; it is linked to not just overall literacy but the ability to recognize, process, integrate, and act on information from a multitude of sources, and this can allow people to make decisions concerning their healthcare and disease prevention. Children are considered health literate once they understand how to achieve health and well-being by obtaining certain attributes as personal hygiene, emotional stability, enjoyment in school life, and the ability to cope with various circumstances [6, 7]. Improving overall literacy is a critical part of achieving adequate HL; this starts in the elementary school level. In the Unites States, approximately 21–23% of adults read at the lowest reading level, approximately fifth grade or lower [8]. This is a major barrier to achieving adequate HL as many materials including prescriptions, patient instructions, and information on diseases or procedures are written at a much higher reading level.

Several specific attributes were identified that impact the development of HL. Nutbeam breaks these down into several attributes [3]. Cognitive skills include information which is required for understanding content and integrating what is presented. Basic health skills include comprehension of instructions such as in prescriptions or basic numerical concepts. Appraisal and critical thinking allow people to evaluate and interpret what is being presented and then formulate questions or discussions to make sound decisions.

Behavioral attributes include information seeking, curiosity, application of the information received, communication, and self-regulation. These are higher order skills that typically evolve with experience and interactions with the healthcare system [3, 5]. Due to the constant acquisition of knowledge, HL is considered to be an evolving process that is developed and nurtured during the life course [5].

Rababah et al. looked at overall HL in college students. The results of this study showed that college students' health literacy is strongly influenced by demographic characteristics. They utilized a health literacy questionnaire and collected sociodemographic data to identify levels of HL which were found to be lower than previously reported. They also found gender, age, smoking status, and field of study had a statistically significant impact on the results. They felt these results could be used to guide future investigation on the effectiveness of tailored interventional programs to improve college students' health literacy. They also hypothesized that the disparity in health literacy based on the field of study provides promising information regarding the usefulness of interprofessional education in optimizing the health outcomes of college students [9].

A study of younger children done in 2020 by Fretian noted that motivation to learn something new about health and a supportive environment in which health-promoting behaviors are endorsed could improve the health literacy of children [10]. Starting the process as early as possible seems to have a beneficial effect on overall HL and the attributes discussed above. The benefits are enormous with more ownership of one's health and outcomes, better understanding of disease prevention, and a healthier population. Stated another way by Borzekowski, the intermediate- and long-term outcomes of HL refer to the promotion of personal health and health outcomes, such as reduction of health risks and the improvement of one's quality of life or living conditions [11].

Measurement of Health Literacy

Several measures exist to assess health literacy at the individual and population level. These measures vary in content and intention, but none are considered comprehensive. The most widely used clinical measures include the Rapid Estimate of Adult Literacy in Medicine (REALM), which tests the ability to read and pronounce a list of words, and the Test of Functional Health Literacy in Adults (TOFHLA), which tests reading comprehension and numeracy. Often used is the Newest Vital Sign (NVS) test which is designed to be a quick clinical screening HL instrument. At the population level, proxy measures of health literacy have been derived from national surveys of literacy that use health-related materials. All the presently available measures of health literacy have focused primarily upon measuring reading, comprehension, and numeracy skills; however, the concept of health literacy is much broader than literacy skills alone. The Health Literacy Toolshed website houses a comprehensive listing of health literacy measures available to clinicians and researchers in this area (https://healthliteracy.bu.edu) [12–15].

Liu conducted a systematic review of the different HL measurement instruments and found that all tools for monitoring health literacy adopted a questionnaire approach. Self-reported monitoring and measurement tools for health literacy are by nature subjective, and results may not be readily interpretable or accurate. For data collection and participant feedback, they suggested that other methods should be combined along with these subjective measures, such as interviews and observations, to increase the authenticity and objectivity of the data [16]. Self-reported measures of HL typically cover health-related knowledge, attitudes, motivation, behavioral intentions, personal skills, and self-efficacy [3, 4]. There may also be a sociodemographic component to these in addition to a basic overall literacy evaluation. The ideal method of measuring HL has not been elucidated; however, a multifaceted approach seems to have the most promise.

Implications of Low Health Literacy

Patient Level

HL has significant individual implications on overall health and utilization of the healthcare system. In general, individuals with limited literacy have less knowledge about their health problems, more hospitalizations, higher healthcare costs, and poorer health status than those with adequate literacy. The relation between limited overall literacy and these factors is consistent across a multitude of studies and persists even after adjusting for confounding sociodemographic variables [2, 17, 18].

A large area where HL plays a critical role is in medication safety. Several studies found that when patients and caretakers have low health literacy, they are at disproportionate risk of difficulty with deciphering medication instructions including dosing, proper storage, and timing of the medicine including any food restrictions [19]. This can cause challenges with improper treatment, under- or overdosing, and medication interactions leading to adverse events. Additionally in surgical patients, low HL was associated with non-adherence to preoperative and/or discharge instructions as well as poor comprehension of surgical procedures [20, 21]. Multiple studies have shown that the informed consent process is flawed and many patients or families do not understand either the procedures or the associated risks of those procedures despite verbal and written explanations [21, 22]. These findings are important because recent studies are beginning to link low HL to poor surgical outcomes, which suggests an opportunity for interventions.

Social determinants of health (SDH) are described in literature as showing significant influence on the HL of children and adolescents, namely, sex, cognitive characteristics, eating habits, family structure and models, school characteristics, school environment, and parents' conditions [23]. Frequent healthcare-related interactions are also influential in the HL of children and families. Interestingly, other studies did not show as much impact of race or ethnicity on health disparities or HL [24]. Mantwill identified a need for more rigorous longitudinal studies along with the need for choosing an appropriate reference group for comparisons [24].

There are a few studies that explored communicative or critical HL in adolescents and young adults (AYAs). Poorer health literacy in AYAs was associated with adverse health outcomes, such as obesity and smoking. For AYAs with a chronic illness, there were mixed findings between level of HL and medication adherence [25].

Interventions targeted at the individual to improve overall HL have been shown to impact overall health-related outcomes. Negative outcomes are clearly linked to lower HL in a variety of areas including medication adherence, surgical outcomes, and management of chronic health conditions.

Health System

Poor HL has been shown to increase health system burden including inpatient length of stay, emergency department (ED) utilization, and readmissions. An exploratory study by Baker in 1998 suggested that patients' reading ability is independently associated with their risk of hospitalization. Patients with inadequate literacy had more than twice the risk of being hospitalized during 1994 and 1995. They noted that patients with poor reading ability may have more difficulty understanding oral instructions because of limited vocabulary or difficulty following complex sentence structure. This could also impact the ability to change their behavior based on new information given. Low HL has a direct impact on provider-patient communication and health behaviors which impacts the risk of hospital admission but may not be directly related just to reading ability [17].

Since children rely on their parent or guardian for their healthcare, their outcome depends largely on how easy the hospital makes it for them to understand and act on information provided. This can impact follow-up care as well as specific instructions regarding medication or activity levels. Lack of attention to HL issues has the potential to create a patient safety risk. Glick states, "Each time an instruction is misunderstood, a medicine is not taken, or an appointment is not kept is a patient safety event, that is, an event that has the potential to lead to a worse patient outcome" [26]. One example cited was parents who believe their child is in pain are found to be less likely to understand information provided during encounters with the healthcare team. Throughout the hospitalization and at the time of hospital discharge, parents are often sleep deprived and are experiencing high levels of stress and fear related to their child's prognosis, which can interfere with their ability to function at their normal level of health literacy. Given that HL is dynamic and not static, a "state" rather than a "trait," healthcare providers should consider all individuals to be at risk for limited HL [26]. This is taking into account the distractions surrounding a hospitalization including emotional, physical, and financial stress which will often times cloud clear thought and comprehension.

Several studies looked at the impact of low HL in the ED setting. Low HL has been correlated with non-emergent utilization of ED services due to difficulty navigating outpatient appointments or the perception that the situation is worse than it is clinically. Other factors that contribute to nonurgent ED use in children include low socioeconomic status, lower educational attainment, quality of primary care and availability, and limited ability of parents to accurately judge the urgency of the condition [27, 28]. May found over half the children presenting to the ED are for nonurgent issues such as viral upper respiratory infections, viral gastroenteritis, rash, and fever [27].

Some of the challenges arise when there is a mismatch between what healthcare providers assume regarding the patient or parent's HL and what is understood by the patient/family. A large part of this is lack of training in these specific communication methods and lack of time to adequately assess how well the communication is understood and interpreted. Studies have shown that not only do physicians have difficulty identifying caregivers or patients with limited health literacy, but pediatricians specifically feel they have inadequate communication skills and time to meet the needs of these caregivers [29]. Medical trainees also perceive that they do not receive adequate training to feel confident in communicating with patients and caregivers with low health literacy [29].

Since communication is vital to convey the appropriate information regarding the health-related problem, treatment plan, and prognosis and address patients' specific needs, it is imperative for the health system to play a role in improving the intelligibility of the materials given regarding these needs. Role playing with trainees may be a method to help ensure information is conveyed and appropriately received and understood. This concept will also elevate the trainees' awareness of the problem and hopefully "pay it forward" by teaching skills that are useful when they are in practice independently. Additionally, implementing some of the HL measurement tools at time of admission or in the ED can help guide the level of complexity that takes place in the discussion with patients and families.

Economy

Quite a few studies have been done showing the impact of low HL on healthcare costs. These have been examined both at the system level and at the patient level. Vernon found that publicly funded insurance such as Medicare and Medicaid as well as uninsured patients have much lower overall or basic HL compared to those with private, military, or employer-provided insurance [30]. This study used data from the National Assessment of Adult Literacy Survey in 2003 and estimated overall costs of low and very low HL to range from $106 billion to $238 billion annually representing 7–17% of US healthcare expenditures [30]. They estimated addressing this disparity could save enough to provide insurance for every uninsured American. Long-term estimates of the cost to the system are in the trillion dollar range [30].

Other studies [2, 30] assessed additional costs due to limited HL on the patient level in selected populations. The amount of additional healthcare expenditures with limited HL compared to a reference group with adequate HL is in a range of $143–7798 per person per year. Persons with low HL also showed a slightly increased use of inpatient and emergency room services (difference in probability: 0.05; 95% CI: 0.00–0.10) and consumed an inefficient mix of healthcare services such as utilization of higher levels of care for low acuity problems [4, 30]. This same study also estimated at 3–5% increased total cost per year due to low HL [4]. One systematic review in 2005 assessed studies that examined the prevalence of limited HL specifically related to US healthcare or health services inquiries. The pooled weighted prevalence in the United States was 26% for low HL and 20% for marginal HL specifically associated with education, ethnicity, and age [31].

Weiss looked at the Arizona Medicaid population to identify factors that increased healthcare-related costs. They evaluated literacy in both English and Spanish and found a large difference in those who had lower than a third grade reading level and those who were above fourth grade. This was independent of sociodemographic factors. The key finding of this study is that persons with low literacy skills generate higher charges for healthcare than do persons with better reading skills. The difference was statistically significant and clinically meaningful. It supports results of other research, which has found that persons with limited literacy skills have poorer health status, are more apt to be hospitalized, and make more visits to emergency rooms than their more literate counterparts [2]. Other analyses have suggested that excess hospitalizations and other ramifications of limited literacy cost the US healthcare system between $50 billion and $73 billion per year [2, 27, 30]. In regard to children, low parent health literacy has been correlated with less health knowledge, confusion about medications, increased preventable emergency room visits, and 30-day readmissions with an estimated cost ranging from $50 billion to $240 billion per year [8, 30, 32].

These costs can be mitigated by a policy to improve overall HL. Implementation of programs to boost HL has the potential to decrease overall health-related costs both at the system and individual level while improving the overall health of the population. With physician and nursing shortages looming, programs that can decrease inappropriate utilization of services, improve access to primary care and insurance, and promote preventative care all are strengthened if they include a more focused plan to bolster HL overall.

Strategies to Improve Health Literacy

A variety of strategies have been proposed to solve the problems of low HL. Determining whether parents and patients can explain key information by using their own words is an evidence-based technique through which health providers can ensure understanding or identify the need for additional education or support. These strategies include techniques such as "teach-back" where a skill is demonstrated and repeated by the caregiver. Others such as "ask me 3" focus on specific questions such as the following: "What is the problem?" "What do I need to do for my child?" "Why is this important?" The use of supplementary materials such as pictograms or child-friendly written handouts also enhances the educational experience [19]. Additional studies are needed to identify the best practices for teach-back and other communication strategies [3, 19].

Another study specifically looked at medication dosing interventions which included a team member who delivered the intervention consisting of a written, pictogram-based medication instruction sheet, teach-back (caregivers state information taught), and demonstration of dosing with show back (caregivers show how they would draw the liquid medication in the syringe). In this study, the intervention group had statistically fewer dose-related errors [33]. As mentioned earlier, there are fewer studies looking at HL in surgical patients. Some newer studies focused on interventions in HL for surgical patients are emerging [34]. In orthopedics, Choi studied the use of Internet-based pictograph-formatted discharge instructions for older adults after hip replacement surgery and reported that participants found the website easy to use and understand [20, 22, 34].

Even in cases of low overall literacy, some interventions specifically focusing on written materials found that improving these handouts to accommodate for lower reading levels can increase overall health knowledge, and combining good written materials with brief counseling can improve behaviors including adherence [1]. This was also found when combining brief videos and written materials: a crossover study showed improved understanding of outpatient procedures in children and caregivers with either modality although in general the video resource was preferred [35]. In order to intervene in many of these cases, health workers, such as nurses, can use a variety of educational strategies to minimize the influence of low HL such as fostering a bond between the family and the health unit in the region, family counseling, referral to community resources, and others [23, 36].

The stigma society places on illiteracy is one of the primary reasons patients often hide their reading difficulties. Creating a shame-free environment where patients receive help without feeling stigmatized, exposed, or humiliated will require a strong partnership with all active staff in the hospital and healthcare team. Hospital personnel should be better informed about the variety of problems that low literate patients have in different areas in the healthcare setting in order to focus on better communication [8, 17, 37]. When discussing risks of interventions, it is critical to avoid misperception and confusion; therefore, attention should be paid to neutral framing and consistent communication terminology [38].

The ultimate aim of HL interventions is to bring about behavior change in order to make an individual/agent/organization behave in a health literate way. In recent years, we can see the behavior change field has developed a considerable number of frameworks, theories, components, and techniques. A review of the impact of interventions on HL started out asking if these activities impacted behavior change, but it also has become apparent that HL interventions can not only influence change but could also learn more from the emerging field of behavior change theory [39].

It is clear there is still much work to be done both in terms of determining best practices healthcare systems and practitioners can use to improve individual and population HL and evaluating how well these interventions affect these changes. In addition, since HL is an evolutionary process, these interventions need to be repeated and reinforced so that the impact is not fleeting. Incorporating use of these educational techniques by healthcare providers into their medical or nursing education is another important factor to create an environment that recognizes and addresses the issues related to low HL and makes an effort to improve it.

Special Considerations

Young Children

Preschool-age children and children from households with low overall literacy are especially vulnerable. These parents may have a multitude of challenges including financial insecurity, child care difficulties, or navigating a single parent household. When young children need to access the healthcare system, this can be an overwhelming process for these parents especially those who have low educational attainment and reading comprehension skills.

As noted previously, HL is a growing problem for Americans, with studies reporting as many as 90 million adults have a limited understanding of basic health information and services. Half of all parents have difficulty reading and understanding patient education materials, and many struggle to comprehend medical advice that is critical to the care of their child [6, 7, 38, 40]. Since HL is understood as a variable construct that is acquired in a lifelong learning process starting in early childhood, targeting children and young people with health literacy interventions can help promoting healthy behaviors and ameliorate future health risks [5, 40, 41].

The impact of low HL is apparent in parental acquisition of knowledge, attitudes, and behaviors, as well as child health outcomes in areas of disease prevention, acute illness care, and chronic illness care. The effect of low health literacy is wide-ranging, including poor nutrition knowledge and behaviors, higher obesity rates, medication errors, increased emergency department use, and poor asthma management, understanding, and outcomes [28, 42]. The shame and embarrassment felt by some low literate patients or parents can pose an important psychological barrier to asking for help or requesting low literate materials, even when they are available [37]. Interventions such as "ask me 3" are beneficial in these situations [19]. This intervention centers on three critical questions: "what is my child's main problem", "what do I need to do for my child" and "why is it important for me to do for my child". These questions center the discussion on the child and help the parent/caregiver understand their role and the purpose of the treatment plan.

Medication errors are a frequent result of poor HL and miscommunication. Math skills may be needed to accurately measure liquid medications for proper dosing. Most pediatric medications are weight-based dosing, and inadequate communication between caregivers and clinicians at hospital discharge has been shown to contribute to medication dosing errors in children [33]. In situations requiring an intervention or a procedure, where parents need to consider the benefits and harms of diagnostic or treatment options, these considerations are critical to allow for true "shared decision-making" and assessment of potential risks [38].

Careful attention has to be given to these caregivers since the young child is unable to self-advocate or understand what is happening. These situations are already scary for the parents, and having a framework to navigate their healthcare journey and explain it to the child in an appropriate manner requires extra attention from the entire healthcare team.

Special Needs Populations

Similar to young children, children with special healthcare needs and their families are candidates for enhanced HL-related strategies, especially those designed to promote self-management of chronic conditions [19]. Parents of children with chronic medical needs often transfer self-care responsibilities when their child is between the ages of 11 and 15 years if they are able to do so. Oftentimes adolescents do not implement the necessary level of self-care activities when the transfer of care occurs, which results in poorer health outcomes [1]. Materials and education designed to empower adolescents with chronic health conditions can be beneficial to improve their ability to self-advocate and avoid negative behaviors [25, 28].

Children with special healthcare needs (CSHCN) are defined by the Maternal and Child Health Bureau as those who have or are at increased risk for a chronic physical, developmental, behavioral, or emotional condition(s) and require healthcare services beyond that required by children generally. It is estimated that between 13% and 18% of children in the United States are CSHCN and their diagnoses can encompass a wide range of pediatric diagnoses [43]. Among children's health expenditures, CSHCN account for between 40% and 70% of all healthcare expenditures among children, and CSHCN often have multiple providers, complex treatment regimens, and high financial burden to the family, including out-of-pocket costs [43, 44]. Especially in CSHCN instances, limited parental health literacy has been linked with increased perceived barriers to access care and negative parental perceptions of their own ability to care for chronic illness [29].

Utilization of team-based resources, including child life specialists, nurse navigators, case managers, and social workers, within the healthcare setting can simplify some of the challenges these parents and children face. The ability for a parent to have a single point of contact when dealing with multiple appointments, admissions, and procedures can minimize the stress associated with access for these children, and these additional resources can improve the entire family's HL by careful attention to communication about the child's needs and care.

Cultural and Language Barriers

There is a paucity of studies looking specifically at language and cultural implications.

The study from the Arizona Medicaid population found that those patients from low socioeconomic status backgrounds, those with low educational attainment, racial/ethnic minority groups, and non-English speakers are disproportionately affected by limited HL [2, 26]. The use of interpreter services helped with communication but did little to affect the overall HL of the non-English-speaking patient [2, 17]. Among hand surgery patients, limited HL significantly affected native Spanish-speaking patients (100%) versus native English-speaking patients (33%) [20]. There is room for more focus on HL in patients whose primary language is not the same as the country they are residing.

A German study looking at HL in children did not find a difference between those who spoke German exclusively and multilingual families; however, they did not address non-German-speaking households in this study [10]. Providing supplementary written or video information in the patient's native language may help mitigate this aspect of language barriers and lower HL.

Impact of the Internet, Social Media, and Technology

With the emergence of wearable health technology and readily accessible websites containing a variety of health information, the influence of technology cannot be underestimated. HL is even more important in the proliferation of misinformation or inaccurate information in the popular media and online.

A study looking at the use of health information technology (HIT) such as wearables and fitness trackers found adequate versus less than adequate health literacy was significantly associated with the use of fitness apps ($P = 0.02$), nutrition apps ($P < 0.001$), activity trackers ($P < 0.001$), and patient portals ($P < 0.001$). Additionally, greater health literacy was significantly associated with greater perceived ease of use and perceived usefulness across all HIT tools after controlling for demographics such as age [45].

Many resources are becoming more available to the general public with the increase in media reports and rapid diffusion of the Internet. Thus, patients' own skills in finding and applying information about health issues may have a substantial impact on their future well-being [46, 47]. Rapid diffusion of Internet technology within the public sphere has placed an unprecedented amount of health information within reach of general consumers. Overall estimates suggest that almost two thirds, or 63.7%, of adults online looked for some type of health or medical information either for themselves or for someone else through the Internet. The use of the Internet for health or medical information was generally more common among persons who were younger than 65 years, women, those who were white or other race (e.g., Asian), and those who had higher levels of education and income [47].

The use of digital media to obtain health information is presently more common among people who are young, educated, and wealthy [3, 48]. Ensuring accuracy of information and helping patients navigate the wide range of resources available add another layer of complexity to an already challenging problem. Patients frequently bring questions or printouts from websites to their appointments to ask about a variety of health conditions or treatments, and the healthcare team needs to be able to adequately address these questions in a way that makes the information meaningful to the patient and family. This may require a general anatomic or physiologic discussion to frame their question around and allow them time to process the new information provided.

Wrap-Up

The issue of HL requires a deeper understanding of the factors that influence HL development, the ways HL is measured, and how different interventions can be used to impact change. Understanding where the patient is from a HL standpoint may take some time and effort but will then allow the healthcare team to positively impact their interactions with the system and possibly prevent less than desirable outcomes. Utilization of resources including team-based care, especially in complex situations or in special needs patients, the patient portal, and other teaching techniques can drastically improve the overall costs of care as well as the health of the population. These methods need to be taught at the provider training level and reinforced throughout each patient encounter to become part of the treatment algorithm. Empowering patients to understand and be able to think critically about their health-related conditions assures more engagement and buy-in from the patient about taking ownership of their health.

Key Takeaways

– Health literacy is critical to achieve better overall outcomes.

- Low health literacy leads to higher costs, poorer results, frequent utilization of higher levels of care such as ED, or hospital admission.
- Healthcare providers often overestimate the health literacy of the patient and family.
- Low health literacy is a large factor in the social determinants of health independent of sociodemographic factors.
- Improving health literacy in families and patients provides the best opportunities for communication of medically relevant information and patient-centered care.
- Many interventions are proven to help but require time and team training to implement.

References

1. DeWalt DA, Hink A. Health literacy and child health outcomes: a systematic review of the literature. Pediatrics. 2009;124(Supplement 3):S265–74.
2. Weiss BD, Palmer R. Relationship between health care costs and very low literacy skills in a medically needy and indigent Medicaid population. J Am Board Fam Pract. 2004;17(1):44–7. In Eng. https://doi.org/10.3122/jabfm.17.1.44.
3. Nutbeam D, Lloyd JE. Understanding and responding to health literacy as a social determinant of health. Annu Rev Public Health. 2021;42:159–73. In eng. https://doi.org/10.1146/annurev-publhealth-090419-102529.
4. Eichler K, Wieser S, Brügger U. The costs of limited health literacy: a systematic review. Int J Public Health. 2009;54:313–24. https://pmc.ncbi.nlm.nih.gov/articles/PMC3785182/pdf/38_2009_Article_58.pdf
5. Bröder J, Okan O, Bauer U, et al. Health literacy in childhood and youth: a systematic review of definitions and models. BMC Public Health. 2017;17(1):361. In eng. https://doi.org/10.1186/s12889-017-4267-y.
6. Vaillancourt R, Cameron JD. Health literacy for children and families. Br J Clin Pharmacol. 2022;88(10):4328–36. In eng. https://doi.org/10.1111/bcp.14948.
7. Van Boxtel W, Jerković-Ćosić K, Schoonmade LJ, Chinapaw MJM. Health literacy in the context of child health promotion: a scoping review of conceptualizations and descriptions. BMC Public Health. 2024;24(1):808. In eng. https://doi.org/10.1186/s12889-024-17955-7.

8. Safeer RS, Keenan J. Health literacy: the gap between physicians and patients. Am Fam Physician. 2005;72(3):463–8. https://www.aafp.org/pubs/afp/issues/2005/0801/p463.pdf
9. Rababah JA, Al-Hammouri MM, Drew BL, Aldalaykeh M. Health literacy: exploring disparities among college students. BMC Public Health. 2019;19(1):1401. In eng. https://doi.org/10.1186/s12889-019-7781-2.
10. Fretian A, Bollweg TM, Okan O, Pinheiro P, Bauer U. Exploring associated factors of subjective health literacy in school-aged children. Int J Environ Res Public Health. 2020;17(5) In eng https://doi.org/10.3390/ijerph17051720.
11. Borzekowski D. Considering children and health literacy: a theoretical approach. Pediatrics. 2009;124:S282–8.
12. Buchbinder R, Batterham R, Ciciriello S, et al. Health literacy: what is it and why is it important to measure? J Rheumatol. 2011;38(8):1791–7. https://www.jrheum.org/content/jrheum/38/8/1791.full.pdf
13. Parker RM, Baker DW, Williams MV, Nurss JR. The test of functional health literacy in adults: a new instrument for measuring patients' literacy skills. J Gen Intern Med. 1995;10(10):537–41. In eng. https://doi.org/10.1007/bf02640361.
14. Weiss BD, Mays MZ, Martz W, et al. Quick assessment of literacy in primary care: the newest vital sign. Ann Fam Med. 2005;3(6):514–22. In eng. https://doi.org/10.1370/afm.405.
15. Nguyen TH, Paasche-Orlow MK, McCormack LA. The state of the science of health literacy measurement. Stud Health Technol Inform. 2017;240:17–33. In eng
16. Liu H, Zeng H, Shen Y, et al. Assessment tools for health literacy among the general population: a systematic review. Int J Environ Res Public Health. 2018;15(8) In eng https://doi.org/10.3390/ijerph15081711.
17. Baker DW, Parker RM, Williams MV, Clark WS. Health literacy and the risk of hospital admission. J Gen Intern Med. 1998;13(12):791–8. https://pmc.ncbi.nlm.nih.gov/articles/PMC1497036/pdf/jgi_242.pdf
18. Morrison AK, Glick A, Yin HS. Health literacy: implications for child health. Pediatr Rev. 2019;40(6):263–77. https://publications.aap.org/pediatricsinreview/article-abstract/40/6/263/35293/Health-Literacy-Implications-for-Child-Health?redirectedFrom=fulltext
19. Abrams MA, Klass P, Dreyer BP. Health literacy and children: recommendations for action. Pediatrics. 2009;124(Supplement 3):S327–31. https://doi.org/10.1542/peds.2009-1162I.
20. Chang ME, Baker SJ, Dos Santos Marques IC, et al. Health literacy in surgery. Health Lit Res Pract. 2020;4(1):e46–65. In eng. https://doi.org/10.3928/24748307-20191121-01.
21. De Oliveira GS Jr, McCarthy RJ, Wolf MS, Holl J. The impact of health literacy in the care of surgical patients: a qualitative systematic review. BMC Surg. 2015;15:86. In eng. https://doi.org/10.1186/s12893-015-0073-6.

22. Kampouroglou G, Velonaki VS, Pavlopoulou ID, Fildissis G, Tsoumakas K. Parental health literacy in the pediatric surgical setting. Chirurgia (Bucur). 2019;114(3):326–30. In eng. https://doi.org/10.21614/chirurgia.114.3.326.
23. Gomes ADS, Santos G, Bastos I, Sales JKD, Perrelli JGA, Frazão C. Social determinants of health literacy in children and adolescents: a scoping review. Rev Gaucha Enferm. 2024;45:e20240002. In eng por. https://doi.org/10.1590/1983-1447.2024.20240002.en.
24. Mantwill S, Monestel-Umaña S, Schulz PJ. The relationship between health literacy and health disparities: a systematic review. PLoS One. 2015;10(12):e0145455. https://pmc.ncbi.nlm.nih.gov/articles/PMC4689381/pdf/pone.0145455.pdf
25. Sansom-Daly UM, Lin M, Robertson EG, et al. Health literacy in adolescents and young adults: an updated review. J Adolesc Young Adult Oncol. 2016;5(2):106–18. In eng. https://doi.org/10.1089/jayao.2015.0059.
26. Glick AF, Brach C, Yin HS, Dreyer BP. Health literacy in the inpatient setting: implications for patient care and patient safety. Pediatr Clin N Am. 2019;66(4):805–26. In eng. https://doi.org/10.1016/j.pcl.2019.03.007.
27. May M, Brousseau DC, Nelson DA, et al. Why parents seek care for acute illness in the clinic or the ED: the role of health literacy. Acad Pediatr. 2018;18(3):289–96. In eng. https://doi.org/10.1016/j.acap.2017.06.010.
28. Morrison AK, Myrvik MP, Brousseau DC, Hoffmann RG, Stanley RM. The relationship between parent health literacy and pediatric emergency department utilization: a systematic review. Acad Pediatr. 2013;13(5):421–9. In eng. https://doi.org/10.1016/j.acap.2013.03.001.
29. Griffeth E, Sharif I, Caldwell A, Townsend Cooper MJR, Tyrrell H, Dunlap M. Health literacy perceptions and knowledge in pediatric continuity practices. Health Lit Res Pract. 2022;6(1):e51–60. In eng. https://doi.org/10.3928/24748307-20220208-01.
30. Vernon JA, Trujillo AJ, Rosenbaum SJ, Debuono BA. Low health literacy: implications for national health policy. 2007.
31. Paasche-Orlow MK, Parker RM, Gazmararian JA, Nielsen-Bohlman LT, Rudd RR. The prevalence of limited health literacy. J Gen Intern Med. 2005;20(2):175–84.
32. Howe CJ, Carsey E, Gamboa J, Zhang Y, Lewis B. Communicate to care: implementing health literacy in a pediatric ears, nose, and throat clinic. Health Lit Res Pract. 2024;8(3):e166–74. In eng. https://doi.org/10.3928/24748307-20240819-02.
33. Carroll AR, Johnson JA, Stassun JC, Greevy RA, Mixon AS, Williams DJ. Health literacy-informed communication to reduce discharge medication errors in hospitalized children: a randomized clinical trial. JAMA Netw Open. 2024;7(1):e2350969. In eng. https://doi.org/10.1001/jamanetworkopen.2023.50969.

34. Choi J. Pictograph-based discharge instructions for low-literate older adults after hip replacement surgery: development and validation. J Gerontol Nurs. 2011;37(11):47–56. In eng. https://doi.org/10.3928/00989134-20110706-03.
35. Del Risco A, Cherches A, Polcaro L, et al. Improving health literacy of elective procedures in pediatric otolaryngology. Otolaryngol Head Neck Surg. 2024;171(2):546–53. https://doi.org/10.1002/ohn.731.
36. Romanova A, Rubinelli S, Diviani N. Improving health and scientific literacy in disadvantaged groups: a scoping review of interventions. Patient Educ Couns. 2024;122:108168. In eng. https://doi.org/10.1016/j.pec.2024.108168.
37. Parikh NS, Parker RM, Nurss JR, Baker DW, Williams MV. Shame and health literacy: the unspoken connection. Patient Educ Couns. 1996;27(1):33–9. https://www.sciencedirect.com/science/article/abs/pii/0738399195007873?via%3Dihub
38. Richter R, Jansen J, Bongaerts I, Damman O, Rademakers J, van der Weijden T. Communication of benefits and harms in shared decision making with patients with limited health literacy: a systematic review of risk communication strategies. Patient Educ Couns. 2023;116:107944. In eng. https://doi.org/10.1016/j.pec.2023.107944.
39. Walters R, Leslie SJ, Polson R, Cusack T, Gorely T. Establishing the efficacy of interventions to improve health literacy and health behaviours: a systematic review. BMC Public Health. 2020;20(1):1040. In eng. https://doi.org/10.1186/s12889-020-08991-0.
40. Cheng TL, Dreyer BP, Jenkins RER. Introduction: child health disparities and health literacy. Pediatrics. 2009;124(Supplement 3):S161–2. https://doi.org/10.1542/peds.2009-1100C.
41. Institute of Medicine Forum on the Science of Health Care Quality I, Implementation, Institute of Medicine Roundtable on Health D, Institute of Medicine Roundtable on Health L. The National Academies collection: reports funded by National Institutes of Health. Toward health equity and patient-centeredness: integrating health literacy, disparities reduction, and quality improvement: workshop summary. Washington: National Academies Press (US). Copyright © 2009, National Academy of Sciences; 2009.
42. von Sommoggy J, Skiba EM, Lander J, Apfelbacher C, Curbach J, Brandstetter S. Health literacy in pediatric consultations on allergy prevention. Health Lit Res Pract. 2024;8(2):e47–61. In eng. https://doi.org/10.3928/24748307-20240320-01.
43. Keim-Malpass J, Letzkus LC, Kennedy C. Parent/caregiver health literacy among children with special health care needs: a systematic review of the literature. BMC Pediatr. 2015;15:92. In eng. https://doi.org/10.1186/s12887-015-0412-x.

44. Newacheck PW, Strickland B, Shonkoff JP, et al. An epidemiologic profile of children with special health care needs. Pediatrics. 1998;102(1 Pt 1):117–23. In eng. https://doi.org/10.1542/peds.102.1.117.
45. Mackert M, Mabry-Flynn A, Champlin S, Donovan EE, Pounders K. Health literacy and health information technology adoption: the potential for a new digital divide. J Med Internet Res. 2016;18(10):e264. (In eng). https://doi.org/10.2196/jmir.6349.
46. Ishikawa H, Yano E. Patient health literacy and participation in the health-care process. Health Expect. 2008;11(2):113–22. https://pmc.ncbi.nlm.nih.gov/articles/PMC5060442/pdf/HEX-11-113.pdf
47. Hesse BW, Nelson DE, Kreps GL, et al. Trust and sources of health information: the impact of the Internet and its implications for health care providers: findings from the first Health Information National Trends Survey. Arch Intern Med. 2005;165(22):2618–24. (In eng. https://doi.org/10.1001/archinte.165.22.2618.
48. Smith B, Magnani JW. New technologies, new disparities: the intersection of electronic health and digital health literacy. Int J Cardiol. 2019;292:280–2. In eng. https://doi.org/10.1016/j.ijcard.2019.05.066.

Language Barriers in the Management of Patients

5

Ana-Maria Fernandez

The Merriam-Webster dictionary defines "communication" as "a process by which information is exchanged between individuals through a common system of symbols, signs, or behavior" [1]. However, in order to establish and maintain any kind of relationship, it is vital to not just attempt to communicate but to make sure that the communication is effective. There are several available definitions of *effective communication*. They all have slightly different wording depending on the field to which you are specifically referring, but they all have one aspect in common: it is not enough to send a message using the same symbols, signs, or behavior. It is critical that the message be received, and by this it is meant that the information sent *must convey the meaning that the sender intended*. In the field of healthcare, effective communication is imperative. Without it, the entire process of health evaluation and problem management is placed at risk, and this risk can profoundly affect people's lives. This chapter is dedicated to evaluating the effect of a very important barrier in the process of effective communication in healthcare: that of language discor-

A.-M. Fernandez (✉)
Duke Pediatric Plastic and Oral Maxillofacial Surgery,
Durham, NC, USA
e-mail: Ana-maria.fernandez@duke.edu

E. Raynor (ed.), *Managing Challenging Patients and Families in Health Care Settings*, https://doi.org/10.1007/978-3-032-10492-2_5

dance. What happens when the member of the healthcare team and the patient and their family speak a different language? This is an issue that impacts the very definition of communication we discussed previously: How do you manage communication about someone's health when you *do not* share the same symbols or signs?

After 23 years working as a nurse and nurse practitioner in different specialties and locations, I have learned a number of key lessons. One of these is that **the healthcare field already has a particular language onto itself**. The field of medicine uses language that is not universally understood, and even among its own members, there can be miscommunication. This means that when we communicate with patients and their families, people who are not in the medical field, we are already speaking to them with terms that they are not familiar with. This presents one language barrier. Then we add the fact that when you are speaking to people about their or their loved one's health, there is a level of anxiety, which can also alter the ability to receive that information [2]. These two points on their own support that talking about health is challenging. If we add language discordance to this situation, meaning that the provider or healthcare worker is not communicating in the same language as the patient and/or their family, then we find ourselves in a very complicated situation.

In healthcare, we rely on effective communication for the entirety of the process with the patient. In a well visit, we must learn about a patient's health history, their family history, the medications/supplements that they are taking, their surgical history, any possible allergies, and any concerns they may have. In a problem-focused visit, we must be able to understand their symptoms, when they started, how they have changed, any interventions that may have been done in the past to help manage an issue, and family history (to name a few). If any of these pieces of information are not accurate or are misunderstood, it could alter our differential diagnosis and subsequently affect the tests we order in order to further investigate an issue [3–5].

As providers, we then have to ask questions to clarify information and narrow things down. We also have to explain to the patient what the examination will entail, what tests we are ordering and why, and what they need to do to obtain said tests. We will then have to speak to them about the results of the tests, what they mean to their immediate- and long-term future, and what interventions may follow such as medications, procedures, surgeries, or any other therapeutic options. Misunderstanding of this information can lead to mistakes in medication dosing, lack of follow-through with treatment, and interruption in follow-up management, among other issues.

Furthermore, the disruption that a language barrier has on the entire healthcare process doesn't only affect the health of the patient. It also has a profound impact on the provider trying to take care of the patient, and it directly affects the healthcare system as a whole. According to the 2019 US Census Bureau, 67 million people in the United States speak a language other than English at home. According to the same census, about 8% of the US population (roughly 5.5 million people) speaks English less than very well and are considered to have "low English proficiency" (LEP) [6, 7].

Given the extensive consequences of the language barrier in healthcare and the very large portion of the US population that is affected by this issue, it should then be a very high priority for us to make sure that the language barriers between us and our patients are diminished as much as is possible.

Impact on the Patient/Family

A baby girl (BG) was born to Hispanic parents who immigrated from Central America. Shortly after birth, she was diagnosed with cystic fibrosis. Due to the condition being rare and the "normal" appearance of the baby, the family struggled to understand or accept the reality of the condition. Despite the use of interpreters on most of the encounters throughout her medical journey, the family failed to understand the severity of her disease. Pulmonary toilet routines were done sporadically if at all given that she "didn't look sick." Medications were not given regularly due to misunderstanding of the importance of preventive measures in giving

her lungs the best chance at health. The family missed appointments due to difficulties with communication (didn't know she had the appointment) and the family's lack of resources. Mom does not drive, and dad works all day. Mom was unable to secure rides for all the necessary medical visits. BG is now 15 years old and sadly has a lung function of about 22%. She has now developed diabetes, and because of her history of poor compliance throughout the years, she is not a candidate for lung transplant. BG now has a younger sibling who was also diagnosed with CF, but given BG's bad health outcomes, the family now doesn't trust the medical providers, and so her prognosis is likely poor as well.

The language barrier is not the only factor affecting the situation described above. There definitely are cultural factors that impacted the parents' behavior (cultural barriers will be discussed in another chapter). However, it is undeniable that health education when the baby was initially diagnosed needed to have been much more effective. The parents' lack of understanding of the chronic and insidious nature of the disease was the underlying issue that led to their lack of compliance and in the end their child's poor health outcomes and the denial of the possibly life-saving option of a lung transplant. Decreased health education is a known issue with language barriers [8], and its long-term effects can be devastating. Misunderstanding of the critical information about the condition also led to lack of compliance with the treatment. This is an issue that is also frequently seen in the low English proficiency (LEP) population [9]. Lack of understanding of the condition itself, the actual instructions for the treatment, or the reasons for the treatment to be done led to either insufficient, ineffective, or even lack of treatment all together.

A 9-year-old LEP patient is followed by pediatric endocrinology. She is on a specific dose of medication previous to her appointment. During the appointment, thyroid levels are drawn in order to evaluate the effectiveness of the dose. When the results come back (after the patient has gone home), the levels are not where the endocrinologist would like. Due to this, the dose for the medication is changed, and a new medication is sent to the pharmacy. A nurse calls the family with

the information but leaves a message on their phone voicemail as she is unable to reach the family. At the follow-up 3 months later, when the patient is seen, the doctor asks how the patient has been doing with the new dose. The mom looks confused and tells the endocrinologist that she has been giving her the same half tablet she was told to give her at the last appointment because this is what the doctor had told her to do. She did not understand the message left in her voicemail and never realized that the medication given to her at the pharmacy had a new dose and new directions. The child was given the wrong dose of medication for 3 months.

Another known effect of language discordance between a patient and their health team is increased medication errors and subsequent adverse effects to medication [3, 6]. Misunderstanding of medical instructions pertaining to a health diagnosis, taking medication, discharge instructions, postsurgical wound care instructions, etc., leads to increased adverse health events [3, 6, 8, 10]. Knowing this, it is easy to understand why the patient population who has a language barrier with their providers is also at an increased risk of readmission to the hospital [6, 10].

A 46-year-old LEP man tells his wife that he has been having rectal bleeding for 7 days. She confides in her employer who happens to be a healthcare provider and who is also a native Spanish speaker. Her employer strongly advises the wife to take him to the doctor for an evaluation. She explains that this could be a serious issue and that it is always important to deal with things as soon as possible in order to have the best possible outcomes. The wife thanks her employer. The next time they see each other, the employer asks how her husband is doing. She replies that he decided not to go because he always has trouble telling people what is wrong and that he feels fine. The bleeding stopped for a few days and has only come back a few times, so he feels it is getting better and doesn't want to go.

The LEP population seeks care much less frequently than the population that has language concordance with the medical providers [4]. This is because they experience increased stress trying to communicate with their providers, are frequently misunderstood, and feel that the level of interpersonal care is lower [4, 8]. Interpersonal care relates to the patient's perception of how respectfully they are treated, if the provider gave them enough time to explain their reasons for the visit, spent enough time with them, addressed their questions and concerns, and answered them in a way that they understood [8]. Due to their delaying seeing a medical provider sooner, their medical issues can progress and become much more serious, leading to increased ER visits, longer hospitalizations, increased need for surgery, delayed surgery, and poorer health outcomes [4, 6, 8, 9].

To expand on the above point, misunderstanding of history and the details of the patient's present issue leads providers to order erroneous or extra tests and can lead to misdiagnoses [4, 10]. This will result in wrong treatment choices and will not only delay identification of the actual issue but will delay its treatment and can end in the creation of new issues or the worsening of the original problem [3, 4, 10]. By the same token, the language barrier will not only affect the management of acute issues. It will directly affect the treatment of chronic conditions and end-of-life care [4].

Every aspect of a patient's health and their resulting quality of life is impacted by their inability to efficiently and accurately communicate with their healthcare team.

Effects on the Healthcare Provider

I am a bilingual provider. I am fluent in both English and Spanish. This gives me a great advantage given that the LEP Hispanic population is a large percentage of our patients. However, I have also had the opportunity to see patients of other cultural backgrounds who also speak little to no English. In these cases, I have had to rely on either in-person, video, or telephone interpreters to help me communicate with these patients. Regardless of the type of interpreting method utilized, it is undeniable and proven every single time that these visits take at least 50% longer than a visit with a language concordant family. During the time I have been in practice, I have also had the opportunity to speak to multiple colleagues in many different specialties, and they all report that regardless of field and type of visit or even if it is a pediatric, adult, or geriatric patient, interactions with language discordant patients take about twice as long as those with same-language patients. In a healthcare climate where volume of patients seen keeps increasing, it is very understandable that visits that take much longer contribute to increasing provider stress [8].

A pediatric specialist spent over 90 min with a family with an in-person interpreter. Given that they had the interpreter present at this visit, the doctor was able to figure out that the patient was "not responding to the treatment" because the parents had misunderstood directions for medication, had missed several important follow-up visits, and had not done therapies at home. With the help of the interpreter, that doctor had to explain everything again, send new prescriptions, get therapies set up, and involve the social worker to help support the family from that moment on. After an exhausting visit and significant frustration, the provider requested that only one of these kinds of cases be scheduled per morning.

Furthermore, providers identify the inability to effectively communicate with their LEP patients as a significant impediment to the delivery of high-quality healthcare [8]. The example given above and all the factors discussed in the previous section support this. Missed appointments, misinterpreted medication instructions, and noncompliance with therapies and treatments, to name a few things, all render the provider's treatment plan useless. This leads to poor outcomes.

It has also been found that despite best efforts and use of interpreters when available, LEP patients still rate their providers much lower than their language concordant counterparts. These provider ratings could potentially affect performance reviews and financial outcomes that are based on these metrics.

Effects on the Healthcare System

Finally, but not less important, management of the LEP population's health leads to a huge increase in resources and cost for the healthcare system [2, 3]. Research has shown that the LEP population is at risk for increased readmission rates and longer admissions [1, 2, 6]. Lack of communication or inefficient or inaccurate communication leads to increased number of diagnostic tests, increased rates of postsurgical infections, higher risk of medication adverse effects, and inappropriate management of chronic conditions [3, 5, 6, 8, 10]. Supporting families with LEP does not only include the need for interpreters or some interpretation tool. It also involves social work, nursing follow-up, communication with primary care providers (when there is one involved), pharmacists, and other specialties. It requires closer monitoring, more in-depth and repeated education, rescheduling of missed appointments, help with securing transportation, when necessary, etc. All of these efforts translate to significant increase in work hours and monetary compensation for all the extra services involved.

I worked as a primary care pediatric nurse practitioner for 9 years. I had the opportunity to work in rural settings in NC, the south side in Chicago, and inner-city Baltimore and in two other urban setting practices. Due to my bilingual status, my patient population would quickly grow to be heavily made up of LEP Hispanic patients. I absolutely loved taking care of this population, and it was enriching beyond words. However, no matter where I was, I became the only advocate they had. I was seeing 25–30 patients per day and had to do all the documentation after those visits. But I also worked through my lunch hour and spent several hours of my afternoon and evening making calls to schools to speak with principals, teachers, and school nurses. I spoke to therapy services and helped coordinate visits. I reached out to food pantries, charity organizations, and insurance companies trying to secure the needs of my patients and their families. This became my second full-time job and utilized all of my free time. It profoundly impacted the time I had to spend with my family and essentially obliterated any time I had to rest or do any self-care. Pediatric primary care was my first love and the goal I pursued when I started my healthcare career. However, after 9 years, I was completely burnt out and had to switch fields completely. Keep in mind I didn't have the extra time constraint of having to use an interpreter. When the provider isn't bilingual, this issue grows even more significant, and the number of people necessary to provide the services I was providing on my own grows even larger.

Possible Solutions

After reviewing the serious effects of the language barrier in the healthcare field, we should address the possible solutions to this concerning problem. When language is the issue, the solution is any method that could be a communication bridge between the two language discordant parties. Several studies have looked into different options for this. It is obvious, but worth mentioning, that language concordance is the preferred option [6, 8]. This means that an emphasis should be placed in educating healthcare providers in the secondary language that is most prevalent in each country based on their minority populations. In the United States, it would be Spanish, but this may not be the case in the rest of the world. Furthermore, education should focus on medical terminology and language. I was born and raised in Colombia, and Spanish is my first language. However, given that my medical training has all happened in English in the United States, I was not qualified to practice medicine in Spanish or to interpret for others until I finished a 40-hour certification course. This is one of the reasons why family members should also not be used as interpreters [10]. Being bilingual does not guarantee that a person is an appropriate interpreter.

Consider the following example that happened at a pediatric orthopedic clinic: **A resident was involved in the care of a pediatric patient who had fractured their leg and had to be put in a cast. The family was non-bilingual Hispanic. The resident knew some Spanish and told the attending physician that she could give the family the discharge instructions, which included cast care and that the family had to come back in 6 weeks to get the cast taken off. After the resident spoke with them, the parents became very agitated, and a phone interpreter had to be utilized to clarify what had caused their reaction. It was then understood that the resident had told them that they had to come back in 6 weeks to have the *bone* removed instead of the *cast* because she confused the terms for cast and bone in Spanish. The word for bone in Spanish is "hueso." The word for cast is "yeso." They rhyme and are pro-**

nounced very similarly, but the resident's confusion understandably led to absolute panic for the patient and the family.

When language concordance is not a possibility however, an in-person interpreter is the best option, followed by interpreter via video and then an interpreter via audio [6, 8]. Studies have shown that the use of a language interpreter increases the degree of health education as well as access to and delivery of higher quality healthcare. They also increase patient satisfaction and patient show rate to appointments [3].

Unfortunately, not all medical locations can offer language interpreters. Some studies have found that in cases where nothing else is available, free applications such as Google Translate and MediBabble can provide some measure of assistance. However, they are definitely not the best method and provide limited benefits [4, 10].

Finding education resources in the patients' native language and having documents translated at an appropriate reading level can also make a very big difference and diminishes miscommunication [9].

To help diminish the extra burden on the healthcare provider, perhaps adapting the allotted time to see bilingual patients to reflect the extra necessary time it takes to conduct a visit with an interpreter would diminish the stress the provider experiences [2]. Facilitating the ease of that communication will also go a long way to support the provider in their attempt to deliver excellent healthcare to their patients that speak a different language. These interventions will also directly affect and diminish the effects on the healthcare system.

It is undeniable that language discordance is a very significant barrier in the healthcare field and affects not just the health of our language discordant families but the well-being of providers and the healthcare system as a whole. However, I firmly believe that being aware of the specific ways in which it affects the process and being proactive in anticipating these issues will have a positive impact on patients, providers, and the healthcare system.

Key Takeaways

- Effective communication is a vital part of safe, effective, high-quality healthcare.
- Disruption to this process has a very serious effect on the care of the patient and their family, their experience, the healthcare provider who is trying to provide that care, and the healthcare system in which the process is occurring.
- Possible solutions to this very serious problem start at the very beginning of the education process of the provider in the form of courses in medical terminology and conversation in the most common secondary languages spoken in their country.
- When language concordance is not available, the best choices are in-person interpreters, followed by interpreter assistance via video and lastly interpreter assistance via audio/telephone.
- When interpreters are not available, free applications such as Google Translate and MediBabble can provide some measure of assistance.
- Increasing the allotted time the provider has to see patients with low English proficiency will also likely diminish stress and relieve provider burnout.
- Any investment in these interventions will have a direct impact on the healthcare system as a whole as well, diminishing the overall financial burden caused by increased risks, increased number of tests, readmissions, postsurgical complications, etc., that happen as a result of miscommunication due to language barriers.

References

1. https://www.merriam-webster.com/dictionary/communication. Accessed 14 Nov. 2024
2. Robinson O, Vytal K, Cornwell B, Grillon C. The impact of anxiety upon cognition: perspectives from human threat of shock studies. Front Hum Neurosci. 2013;7:1–21.
3. Shamsi H, Almutairi A, Mashrafi S, Kalbani T. Implications of language barriers for healthcare: a systematic review. Omam Med J. 2020;35(2):e122.

4. Moissac D, Bowen S. Impact of language barriers on quality of care and patient safety for official language minority francophones in Canada. J Patient Exp. 2019;6(1):24–32.
5. Cohen A, Rivara F, Marcuse E, McPhillips H, Davis R. Are language barriers associated with serious medical events in hospitalized pediatric patients? Pediatrics. 2005;116(3):575–9.
6. Lopez Vera A, Thomas K, Trinh C, Nausheen F. A case study of the impact of language concordance on patient care, satisfaction, and comfort with sharing sensitive information during. Med Care. 2023;25:1261–9.
7. Dietrich S, Hernandez E. Language use in The United States:2019. 2022. https://www.census.gov/content/dam/Census/library/publications/2022/acs/acs-50.pdf. Accessed 26 Dec 2024.
8. Ngo-Metzger Q, Sorkin D, Phillips R, Greenfield S, Massagli M, Clarridge B, Kaplan S. Providing high quality care for limited English proficient patients: the importance of language concordance and interpreter use. J Gen Intern Med. 2007;22:324–30.
9. Slade S, Sergent S. Language barriers. StatPearls [Internet]. Treasure Island (FL): StatPearls Publishing; 2024. PMID: 29939596.
10. Squires A. Strategies for overcoming language barriers in healthcare. Nurs Manage. 2018;49(4):20–7.

6 Cultural Considerations

Monica Ogunsusi

Introduction

Culture is defined as the beliefs, social norms, and material traits of a racial, religious, or social group. Those of the same culture may share similar sets of attitudes, practices, language, and values. The effect of culture on an individual's identity, behavior, view of the world, and belief system is significant and should be taken into account when providing medical care [1–3].

Cultural awareness is the ability to recognize that individuals from different backgrounds may think, interact, and behave in distinct ways. **Cultural competence** builds upon this understanding and develops ways of interacting with those from differing cultures with sensitivity and respect. While it is not necessary to understand every nuance of each culture to provide effective care, maintaining a general awareness of cultural differences can help guide meaningful interactions. Practicing active listening, remaining open-minded toward experiences different from one's own, extending empathy and compassion, and reflecting on personal

M. Ogunsusi (✉)
Department of Head and Neck Surgery & Communication Sciences, Duke University, Durham, NC, USA
e-mail: Monica.Ogunsusi@duke.edu

E. Raynor (ed.), *Managing Challenging Patients and Families in Health Care Settings*, https://doi.org/10.1007/978-3-032-10492-2_6

biases can aid providers in caring for patients from various backgrounds effectively [3, 4].

Some areas within culture that would be beneficial for healthcare providers to consider include family dynamics, belief systems, social norms, and communication.

Family Dynamics

In western society, individualistic culture predominates [5]. In an **individualistic** society, value is placed on independence, personal advancement, individual choice, self-reliance, and self-actualization. Family units tend to be smaller, with a focus more on the immediate family ties. Parents will place more of an emphasis on children developing autonomy and critical thinking skills. Adolescents and young adults will aim to become financially independent early on and care for themselves. Individuals are encouraged to solve problems on their own [5, 6].

A high prevalence of collectivistic cultures can be found in East Asia, Middle East, throughout Africa, and Latin America [6]. **Collectivist** cultures value social cohesion with emphasis on community, immediate and extended family, interdependence, and tradition. Family units tend to be larger with multiple generations cohabitating. Respect for authority influences parenting styles, and decisions are made as a collective [5, 6].

Understanding these dynamics can be helpful in clinical settings. When discussing medical decision-making with patients, it may be helpful to ask whether including anyone else in the conversation is important to them. For some individiuals, making medical decisions is a personal responsibility alone, while others may prefer to involve family members or loved ones, either by reviewing educational resources together at home with family or by having them present during clinic visits to participate in shared decision-making.

Belief Systems

The care of a patient would be incomplete without consideration of their personal **belief systems**. Many individuals consider their beliefs to be integral to their identity and way of life. In regard to **religion**, patients who identify with a particular religion may use their faith system to guide them in their decision-making. Specific religious practices or traditions may influence how patients and their families engage with the healthcare system [5, 7, 8].

Though not an exhaustive list, a few considerations that relate to patient interactions and healthcare are listed as follows:

Diet

Bottom line: Discuss with patient's dietary restrictions to avoid, when possible, prescribing medications or using surgical devices that conflict with their religious or cultural practices.

Judaism: Jewish patients may follow a strict kosher diet. Pork, certain seafoods, and certain dairy products are a few examples of foods not considered kosher and avoided by those of the Jewish faith. This may have implications with certain ingredients contained with medications. Exceptions are permissible for life-sustaining medications.

Islam: Muslim patients may follow a strict halal diet. Certain foods, such as shellfish and pork, are prohibited. When no other halal alternatives exist, it is permissible for patients to take life-sustaining medication with these prohibited ingredients.

Hinduism: Hindu patients may abstain from beef as well as pork. When no other alternatives exist, it is permissible for patients to take life-sustaining medication with these ingredients.

Health

Bottom line: When recommending medical treatments that may conflict with religious or cultural practices, foster an open discussion with the patient. Avoid judgment, and provide

a clear explanation for risk and benefits of any available alternative options.

Jehovah's Witness: Jehovah's Witnesses have limitations to blood products and generally will not accept blood transfusions.

Various religious groups believe health to be multifactorial, with importance on the mind, body, and soul in relation to one another.

Practices

Bottom line: When possible, seek ways to honor the patient's request.

Islam: Physical contact, including handshakes, is prohibited between genders. Muslims may ask for providers of the same sex to limit contact with the opposite gender.

Sikhism: As a tenet of their faith, hair is not to be cut on any part of the body. This may present a challenge with surgical site preparation. This should be discussed with the patient and, if requested, their spiritual leader when it is necessary to clip hair so the procedure can be performed safely.

Various religious groups partake in fasting from food and drink as a spiritual practice. Exemptions are often made for young children, pregnant and breast-feeding mothers, and those with medical ailments. This practice is important for a healthcare provider to be aware of when counseling patients regarding their health and medications.

Social Norms

Within a given society, **social norms** represent the shared beliefs, values, and behaviors that are deemed acceptable or unacceptable and guide how individuals live and interact with one another.

Behavior

Making direct eye contact can be interpreted different across cultures. In some Native American, Asian, African, Middle Eastern, and Hispanic cultures, direct or prolonged eye contact may be perceived as disrespectful or confrontational. In contrast, within many western cultures, maintaining eye contact is viewed as a sign of respect and active engagement.

Physical contact between opposite genders in some cultures heavily influenced by religious practices has limitations. When interacting with a patient for whom modesty is a significant concern, it is respectful to discuss the examination beforehand, either directly with the patient, or when appropriate, with a male family member or representative. Patients may also request a provider of the same gender be present during the exam or procedure to preserve their sense of modesty and comfort.

Perception of Illness

Perception of illness variess widely across cultures. Different cultures may hold unique views about whether an illness is physical, psychological or "imagined", or spiritual in nature; whether it warrants sympathy the degree of stigma it carries; its perceived causes; and what type of person might be susceptible to it [7]. Understanding a patient's beliefs about illness, including preferred approaches to healing such as medication, traditional remedies, or spiritual practice, can support more holistic and compassionate care. Providing education within this framework and taking time to address concerns are essentials steps in building trust and promoting understanding.

Trust

In cultures where respect for authority figures is an expected social norm, healthcare providers are generally viewed as trusted and reliable sources of guidance [8]. Patients from these backgrounds may heavily rely on the provider to make medical decisions on their behalf and may be less accustomed to participating in a “shared decision-making” model.

Mistrust in the medical system is rooted in historical and ongoing experiences of inequitable treatment, particularly among marginalized communities [9]. Historical references to unethical medical research, well-documented medical discrimination, and systematic inequalities in healthcare access have all contributed to this mistrust [9]. By demonstrating cultural competence and providing care that is both respectful and empathetic, healthcare providers can begin to rebuild trust, especially among historically marginalized communities, including indigenous peoples and incarcerated individuals [9]. Upholding the core ethical principles of beneficence, non-maleficence, and respect is paramount to establishing a productive clinician-patient relationship.

Clinical Scenario
An 8-year-old Hispanic male being seen for sleep apnea is noted to have tonsillar hypertrophy. Adenotonsillectomy is recommended. The parent is concerned that removing tonsils will cause infertility and does not want to proceed with that recommendation. Discussing this in a nonthreatening way with the parent and patient is critical to help them reach understanding about risks of the surgery and that there is no impact on fertility from the procedure. Explaining the role of the tonsils in layperson terms and impact of their removal on the patient's sleep as well as overall health is important for the provider to spend time on. This may require more than one visit to allow for the family to feel reassured about the advice being given and alleviate their fears about adverse impact on fertility in the future.

Communication

Medical interpreters should be offered when interacting with a patient whose preferred language differs from that of the provider. In cultures that place a high value on privacy, some patients may decline interpreter services and instead prefer theuse of a family member who is willing to translate. Considering health literacy levels is especially important in these scenarios, and providers should make every effort to communicate in simple terms and illicit a degree of patient understanding.

Within the English language, there are different vernaculars to take into consideration. African American vernacular English, Chicano English, British English, and Cajun English are a few vernaculars within the English language that a provider may encounter. An phrase in one vernacular may carry a different meaning in another. Asking clarifying questions and avoiding making assumptions when encountering unfamiliar speech patterns can help facilitate understanding between patient and provider.

Conclusion

Providers can deliver more comprehensive, patient-centered care when they take into account a patient's background and culture. Doing somay require more targeted questions to understand how the patient's cultural context influences their perception of illness, treatment options, and medical decision-making. Enhancing' cultural competence significantly improves patient care by fostering trust, improving communication, and promoting better health outcomes.

Key Points

- Culture can have a significant impact on an individual's identity, behavior, and belief system and should be taken into account when providing medical care.
- Recognizing that there will be gaps in a provider's understanding of a patient's cultural background can help the provider guide their open-ended questions. This includes, but is not limited to, family dynamics, belief systems, social norms, and communication.
- Open communication between provider and patient can help foster respect and trust.

References

1. LeDoux J, Mann C, Demoratz M, Young J. Addressing spiritual and religious influences in care delivery. Prof Case Manag. 2019;24(3):142–7. [PubMed]
2. Epner DE, Baile WF. Patient-centered care: the key to cultural competence. Ann Oncol. 2012;23(Suppl 3):33–42. [PubMed]
3. Swihart DL, Yarrarapu SNS, Martin RL. Cultural religious competence in clinical practice. [Updated 2023 Jul 24]. In: StatPearls [Internet]. Treasure Island (FL): StatPearls Publishing; 2025. Available from: https://www.ncbi.nlm.nih.gov/books/NBK493216/
4. Lapinski MK, Rimal RN. An explication of social norms. Commun Theory. 2005;
5. Kemmelmeier M. Cultural orientations in the United States (re)examining differences among ethnic groups. Cross-Cult Psychol. 2001;3(32):348–64.
6. Nickerson C. Individualistic cultures and example behavior. Simply Psychology. 2023. https://www.simplypsychology.org/what-are-individualistic-cultures.html
7. General OOTS. Chapter 2 culture counts: the influence of culture and society on mental health. In: Mental health: culture, race, and ethnicity – NCBI bookshelf; 2001. https://www.ncbi.nlm.nih.gov/books/NBK44249/.
8. Culture-Sensitive Health Care: Middle Eastern-American patients. diversityresources.com. n.d. Retrieved March 30, 2025, from https://www.diversityresources.com/health/me.html
9. Bazargan M, Cobb S, Assari S. Discrimination and medical mistrust in a racially and ethnically diverse sample of California adults. Ann Fam Med. 2021;19(1):4–15. https://doi.org/10.1370/afm.2632.

Ethical Dilemmas

7

Yolanda Troublefield and Eileen Raynor

Introduction

Ethical principles of beneficence, non-maleficence, patient autonomy, and justice are the underpinnings of how medical professionals should approach every patient encounter and think through the recommended care plans using this lens [1]. Fundamentally, each patient has the right to make their own healthcare decisions. Physicians have an obligation to communicate effectively, inform the patient of the risks and benefits of the condition and treatment options, respect the wishes and concerns of the patient, and engage in meaningful discussion to optimize their outcome. Remaining committed to doing the best by the patient, respecting their privacy, maintaining fair treatment, and nondiscrimination are all vital parts of these broader principles [1].

Y. Troublefield
Private Practice, Dartmouth, MA, USA

E. Raynor (✉)
Head and Neck Surgery & Communication Sciences, Duke University Health, Durham, NC, USA
e-mail: eileen.raynor@duke.edu

E. Raynor (ed.), *Managing Challenging Patients and Families in Health Care Settings*, https://doi.org/10.1007/978-3-032-10492-2_7

Diagnostic Dilemmas

Genetic testing is often brought to mind in these cases. Patients may want to know their risk for certain conditions, and testing can sometimes reveal additional mutations that may have long-term or lethal implications such as Huntington's chorea or breast cancer. Additional concerns relate to risk of noncoverage by health insurers or discrimination by employers based on the test results [2]. A case in 1927 highlights this specific issue. A patient and her 7-month-old daughter were labeled as "feebleminded," and Justice Oliver Wendell Holmes upheld a Virginia court ruling on eugenic sterilization, requiring the patient to be sterilized against her wishes. In the 1970s, African American children were required to be tested for sickle cell disease prior to entering school despite sickle cell anemia not being a communicable disease [2]. The introduction of the Health Insurance Portability and Accountability Act (HIPAA) in 1996 barred insurers from using predictive studies as a means of denial of coverage; however, once denied many patients still were unwilling to file a claim for their genetic testing. Other concerns arise regarding disclosure of the information to the patient and whether that should be extended to family who may also be at risk for the condition [2]. By working with genetic counselors who are trained in nondirective techniques where they can uphold patient autonomy and allow for better informed decision-making by the patient, inadvertent disclosures can be avoided. Genetic counselors can also help address additional questions or concerns that the patient may have based on the results of the testing.

Another area this occurs is with incidental findings on imaging studies. A good example is seen when a study was performed for one particular assessment but found to have something else that was not previously suspected. Depending on the risks and the patient's understanding of this new finding, they may undergo a multitude of additional diagnostic tests and treatment which was unanticipated. Several studies have shown that new unexpected pathology can be revealed in up to 75% of PET scans [3]. While the majority of these are benign, there is a small percentage that may have clinical significance. There is no good consensus on how or whether to disclose incidental findings in these studies, and this is even more nebulous when the study is under a research protocol [3, 4]. In cases where an incidental malignancy is identified, there is insufficient data to demonstrate whether there is a reduction in mortality versus overutilization of imaging or other diagnostic tests for surveillance, especially in cases where treatment does not impact overall survival [5].

Treatment Decisions

Frequently, these decisions are centered around end-of-life care or palliative care. While there is more awareness of the need for a living will and a healthcare proxy or power of attorney (POA) to assist in the decision-making process, there can be disagreement among family members and healthcare team providers as to the best way to interpret patient wishes. These decisions may be centered around the use of a feeding tube or tracheostomy, need for intubation, or placement in a long-term care facility. Clarifying the patients' and the families' care goals is paramount as the results of the treatment will have impact beyond the hospitalization [1, 6]. Other situations occur when the treatment decision cannot be supported by resources in the family home. One such example is tracheostomy placement for ventilator dependence in a patient where they do not have access to electricity or clean water. That can put the patient at high risk for morbidity and mortality. In this situation, the discussion around goals of care is paramount: does the family want the patient to come home and potentially die in a familiar environment, or do they want to "do everything" to keep the patient alive regardless of circumstance. Are they willing to place the patient in a long-term care facility, and do they have the financial resources to do so? A clear discussion of the patient's prognosis and risks for additional medical deterioration is also critical to help families understand the impact of their decision [6].

Escalation of Care

This can be the result of a complication from the underlying medical condition or from the treatment itself. Depending again on the risks of further intervention, the patient needs to be informed of what options exist and the risks and benefits to each of those choices. For cases in which the patient is incapacitated due to dementia or other mental conditions, the family, a healthcare proxy, or a guardian ad litem may be needed to help make the necessary decisions for further treatment [7]. An example where the family and patient involvement has been demonstrated to improve clinical outcomes is when there is recognition by the family or patient about deterioration of their condition prompting a rapid response call. Since the nursing staff is not continuously at the bedside, utilizing the families' help in recognizing a change in status can actually allow for faster identification and management of the condition [8]. In some cases, however, communication failure between the patient and the staff can lead to unnecessary escalation, creating a strain on resources [8].

Clinical Scenario

The primary team requested a tracheostomy and gastrostomy for a 19-year-old patient with severe traumatic brain injury after MVC, quadriplegia, and concern for locked-in syndrome. The family has very limited resources, English is not their primary language, and it is unclear how much they understand the patient's long-term overall condition. The consultant team was extremely concerned that the patient will have difficulty accepting the situation they are in.

De-escalation or Withdrawal of Care

In cases where further care efforts are futile such as in brain death or terminal metastatic cancer, decisions such as hospice placement or removal of life support may become necessary. These conversations are often emotionally charged and require extra attention to both verbal and nonverbal cues from the family and other healthcare team members. The decision may need to be revisited if possible, to allow some time to process the presented information. Several guidance documents have been developed to help ICU providers address these situations [9]. Many of these discuss both the ethical and legal issues related to withdrawal or withholding of life support in patients whose conditions are felt to be futile [9]. Futility has been defined in this context as treatment that has no physiologic benefit, failure of three or more vital organs, or incurable disease without potential for palliation or improving functional status [9]. In cases of nonagreement between families/patients and their physicians, the use of a third-party reviewer may be helpful to determine that everything has been done to ensure this is the correct course of action.

Professional Conflicts of Interest

The AMA and specialty professional societies have policies that recommend against treatment of immediate family members as that can post serious ethical problems. Some of the concerns with treating family members relate to feeling pressure to treat conditions not within one's scope of practice, inability to keep accurate records, and challenges regarding continuity of care. Exceptions are typically made for short-term conditions such as an acute illness or in emergency care. Though in general long-term management of family members is not advised, many physicians do write prescriptions such as antibiotics, answer medically relevant questions, and offer advice to family members. Typically, situations that may involve ordering tests, procedures, or care coordination should be left to the patients' actual physician and not the family member [10]. A case highlighting the impact of this dilemma describes a scenario where a cardiothoracic surgeon is called in to take care of an elderly lady with a three-vessel cardiac occlusion necessitating a bypass procedure. The physician comes into the room and realizes it is his mother. He's just out of fellowship and the junior colleague is on call. The case explores several options and the ethical consideration of each one [11]. Ultimately, the least fraught option was having his on-call colleague take over the case and manage his mother's care; however, the situation does demonstrate how the provider may feel obligated to remain involved in the care.

Additionally, entering personal or sexual relationships with patients constitutes a breach of ethical principles and a lack of professionalism. These situations can create moral injury for the patient and the provider and cause the provider serious professional implications from sanctioning to loss of licensure.

Dismissal of the Patient from the Practice

This topic is covered in a different chapter; however, ethical considerations occur specifically regarding abandonment, risk of injury or harm to the patient, or inequitable policies such as decisions whether or not to accept unvaccinated patient into the practice.

There needs to be written policy regarding the criteria used to determine who will be dismissed from the practice, the necessary documentation, the process by which the patient and family is notified of the decision, and a plan for emergency and interim care until another provider is identified who is willing to accept the patient [12, 13].

Summary

Ensuring that all options have been exhausted and that the patient and family understand why the decisions are being made with opportunity for answering questions in a careful and thoughtful way is a critical factor in these very difficult situations. Gathering resources from a variety of specialties and services to aid in this communication can often help mitigate any moral injury that these ethical situations pose.

Clinical Pearls

- Ethical situations require thoughtful consideration of ethical principles: patient autonomy, beneficence, non-maleficence, and justice.
- Utilization of an ethics consult can help with difficult decisions regarding care especially in the ICU setting.
- Maintaining open communication with patients and families, ensuring clear language, and feedback to ensure understanding can resolve many questions regarding care decisions and keep the patient at the center of their care.
- Understanding the laws of the state, hospital policy, and regulations regarding professionalism and ethical standards helps when facing significant challenges in managing care for friends or family.

References

1. Desai MK, Kapadia JD. Medical professionalism and ethics. J Pharmacol Pharmacother. 2022;13(2):113–8.
2. Fulda KG, Lykens K. Ethical issues in predictive genetic testing: a public health perspective. J Med Ethics. 2006;32(3):143–7.
3. Angelis GI, Ockenden K, Meikle SR, Calamante F. Managing incidental findings in total body PET/CT studies: balancing ethical considerations and resource constraints. EJNMMI Rep. 2025;9(1):18.
4. Scott IA, Slavotinek J, Glasziou PP. First do no harm in responding to incidental imaging findings. Med J Aust. 2024;220(1):7–9.
5. Smith-Bindman R. Use of advanced imaging tests and the not-so-incidental harms of incidental findings. JAMA Intern Med. 2018;178(2):227–8.
6. Kuczewski MG, Brubaker L. AMA Journal of Ethics®. 2017.
7. Stivers T, McCabe R. Dueling in the clinic: when patients and providers disagree about healthcare recommendations. Soc Sci Med. 2021;290:114140.
8. Albutt AK, O'Hara JK, Conner MT, Fletcher SJ, Lawton RJ. Is there a role for patients and their relatives in escalating clinical deterioration in hospital? A systematic review. Health Expect. 2017;20(5):818–25.
9. Gedge E, Giacomini M, Cook D. Withholding and withdrawing life support in critical care settings: ethical issues concerning consent. J Med Ethics. 2007;33(4):215–8.

10. Hutchison C, McConnell PC. The ethics of treating family members. Curr Opin Anesthesiol. 2019;32(2):169–73.
11. Kerrigan J, Rovelstad S, Kodner IJ, La Puma J, Keune JD. All in the family: how close is too close? The ethics of treating loved ones. Surgery. 2011;149(3):433–7.
12. Lippman H, Davenport J. Patient dismissal: the right way to do it. J Fam Pract. 2011;60(3)
13. Wicclair M. Dismissing patients for health-based reasons. Camb Q Healthc Ethics. 2013;22(3):308–18. https://www.cambridge.org/core/journals/cambridge-quarterly-of-healthcare-ethics/article/abs/dismissing-patients-for-healthbased-reasons/39BBC05A88BB148E114516FAA9975054

De-escalation Techniques in Healthcare

8

Ashley Milinichik

Introduction

As a healthcare professional, you can likely think of several occasions in which you've encountered a challenging patient situation. Given the sheer number of patients who may seek care at your healthcare institution, it is not surprising that one would encounter a challenging patient or situation on any given day. These common occurrences can lead to stress in the workplace, decreased job satisfaction, and burnout [1]. It is also reasonable to believe that experiencing these difficult situations may interfere with delivering first-rate clinical care and would negatively affect the overall healthcare experience for both the patient and healthcare professional. Teaching de-escalation skills in what can be a high-stress environment such as a healthcare setting may help to keep conflict at bay and result in improved satisfaction levels for all parties. Unfortunately, de-escalation techniques are not regularly emphasized in traditional medical education and training programs [2]. This may suggest that healthcare professionals are not well prepared with the resources they need to navigate difficult

A. Milinichik (✉)
Patient Navigator, Duke University Hospital, Durham, NC, USA
e-mail: Ashley.milinichik@duke.edu

E. Raynor (ed.), *Managing Challenging Patients and Families in Health Care Settings*, https://doi.org/10.1007/978-3-032-10492-2_8

patient interactions. To address this, it is important to first take a closer look at what psychological, social, and systemic factors may be contributing to difficult interactions. We will then explore practical strategies on how to manage complex patient interactions and review de-escalation techniques that can help healthcare professionals in their everyday practice.

Understanding Difficult Patients and Families

As previously mentioned, encountering challenging behaviors in healthcare is a widespread issue. Studies show that in clinical environments such as emergency departments and psychiatric units, up to 92% of staff report verbal aggression, and 52% report physical aggression [1]. Drach-Zahavy et al. indicated that these difficult behaviors may be linked to various factors including but not limited to an individual's "cognitions, beliefs, and expectations" (as cited in [3]). Conflict usually results not from the situation itself but from how interactions or events are perceived [3]. The literature suggests that confirmation bias is a factor that contributes to conflict as individuals tend to focus on information that aligns with their preexisting beliefs and less attention is paid to information that does not align with those beliefs [3]. This bias likely contributes to the aggressive behavior shown by patients and their families and can also influence how healthcare professionals perceive and respond to aggressive behavior [3].

As a healthcare professional, you likely see a broad spectrum of patients as it relates to age, race, gender, medical issues, socioeconomic status, and other demographics. It is no surprise that these same patients also come with unique medical and psychosocial histories, which may include anxiety, mistrust, language barriers, cultural differences, and previous healthcare experiences [4]. All of these factors can have an influence on their interactions with healthcare professionals [4]. The unique histories that these patients bring with them may lead to strain and miscommunication, which can negatively impact the quality of the patient-provider relationship [4]. It is also important to be aware of underlying mental health issues, which can have a significant impact on how people are affected by their environment, particularly in a potentially stressful environment such as healthcare settings. In fact, studies show that nearly 15% of patients are considered "difficult" by their healthcare providers, and those patients are more likely to have mental health disorders, including personality disorders, depression, anxiety, and other mental disorders [5]. Furthermore, patients labeled as difficult are almost two times more likely to have a mental disorder than patients described as non-difficult [6]. Some other factors that may contribute to aggression include delays in care, lack of communication, cognitive challenges, and substance use [1]. Drach-Zahavy et al. explained that if healthcare providers can better identify and understand some of these underlying factors contributing to conflict, they may be better able to adjust their approach with patients and families during high-conflict situations (cited in [3]). This brings us to the topic of de-escalation, an important tool when managing such interactions.

What Is De-escalation?

De-escalation is a concept you have likely heard of, but it should be better defined for healthcare professionals when it comes to caring for difficult patients and families. De-escalation is defined as "a combination of strategies, techniques, and methods aimed at minimizing a patient's agitation and aggression" [7]. De-escalation intends to help stop or prevent the escalation of undesirable behaviors [8]. This method is oftentimes called conflict resolution, verbal de-escalation, or crisis intervention [8]. Even though these other terms are sometimes used interchangeably with de-escalation, it is important to highlight some key differences between them:

- Conflict resolution is "a communication process that is utilized to resolve conflict. It involves the use of negotiation to come to a solution that is agreeable to all parties" [9].
- Verbal de-escalation is described by Hallett and Dickens and Richmond et al. as a method that "involves encouraging the

agitated person to verbalize thoughts, feelings, and problems" to determine the cause of the agitated behavior and to calm the person down (as cited in [9]).

- Crisis intervention is described by Townsend as therapeutic skills used to intervene successfully and safely with individuals in crisis (as cited in [9]). Boyd describes that those in crisis may experience a "debilitating imbalance in one's internal equilibrium caused by a sudden stressor or threat to the self" (as cited in [9]).

Essential Elements of De-escalation Plans

Now that we have outlined the various factors that may influence difficult patient behaviors and have a clear definition of de-escalation, we will identify the elements of de-escalation with examples included. These elements include effective communication, use of nonverbal techniques, control of the environment, awareness of triggers, and team collaboration.

The Importance of Communication in De-escalation

Effective communication is one of the most important tools in your toolbelt when attempting to de-escalate a situation. Key components include active listening, empathy, and listening with a calm attitude [10]. When speaking, it is important to maintain a gentle tone, validate the person's feelings (not their actions), and provide choices when able [10]. When appropriate, validating emotions and providing solutions that can be acted upon can help to reduce frustration and aggression [10]. The main goal in easing a tense situation is to build rapport and establish trust [10].

Example A patient in the waiting room becomes loud and unruly after a long wait to be seen. A healthcare professional may address this patient and situation by stating, "I apologize for the extended delay. I understand it is frustrating to have a long wait to be seen. It is our goal to see you in a timely manner. The team is working hard to see you as soon as possible. I will check on your status and be back with an update soon. In the meantime, can I bring you a water or get you anything to make you more comfortable?"

De-escalation is just as much about nonverbal communication as it is about what is said. Body language can have a significant influence during a difficult encounter. It is important to maintain an open posture, ensure appropriate personal distance, and establish good eye contact [4]. During tense situations, the healthcare professional should try to remain patient, composed, and nonconfrontational, even during a difficult interaction. This will help to improve the immediate situation and can build trust and satisfaction with the patient in the long term [10].

Example A patient is upset and yelling after attempting to check into his appointment and being told that the appointment had been cancelled due to provider illness. The patient states he was not notified of the cancellation until he arrived at the check-in desk. The healthcare professional may approach the patient with an open posture and maintain eye contact at eye level and an appropriate distance. The healthcare professional maintains a calm and composed demeanor while addressing his concerns with empathy.

The Role of Environmental Factors in Promoting De-escalation

It is critical to keep in mind that the environment matters when trying to de-escalate a situation. The Joint Commission emphasizes the need for an environment that supports this effort [7]. Healthcare professionals should aim to find a safe, quiet space that provides privacy when de-escalating a situation [7]. Nursing stations and emergency departments are examples of environments that often have high noise levels such as call bells, alarms, and overhead announcements. These loud environments can exacerbate stress and agitation for many patients. Consider implementing noise-reducing strategies such as reducing overhead announcements, using soft lighting, and having quiet areas readily available. Training staff to control noise levels and respond to call bells in a timely manner can also improve the environment can also improve the environment.

Example An elderly patient is waiting on a stretcher in the hallway of the busy and noisy emergency department. The patient begins to become agitated, groaning in pain, and is seemingly bothered by the recurrent overhead announcements and bright lights. A healthcare professional could work to find a quieter room or space for the patient to wait to see the doctor.

Recognizing Triggers and Signs of Agitation

The ability to identify signs of agitation and understand triggers that lead to aggression is one of the keys to successful de-escalation. Some examples of early signs of agitation include increases in verbal demands, restlessness, and nonverbal signs such as clenching or having a tense posture [11]. Triggers that can lead to these signs of agitation include but are not limited to fear, pain, and loss of control [4]. If healthcare professionals can recognize these signs and triggers, they will be able to intervene in a more timely manner to prevent escalation of conflict [11].

Example A family member starts behaving restlessly, speaking louder, and assuming a tense stance after waiting to see his loved one after a longer than expected surgery. A healthcare professional might approach and say, "I know the surgery lasted longer than you anticipated and it's stressful and frustrating having to wait to see your loved one in the PACU. I will check in to see if the PACU is ready for you. What else can I do for you right now to help you feel more comfortable?"

Collaboration During De-escalation

De-escalation efforts are most effective when it is a joint effort between healthcare team members. Foss Durant, McDermott, Kinney, and Triner described how it is important to remember that "every member of the healthcare team who interacts with a patient plays a role, including doctors, admission clerks, transport staff, dietary staff, housekeeping staff, administrative staff and the business office staff" (as cited in [9]). The healthcare team must be aware of what others in their unit or clinic are doing to de-escalate difficult situations so that they can intervene as necessary, provide consistent messaging, and remain on the same page.

Example A patient's health is rapidly deteriorating in the ICU. Multiple family members are beginning to grow visibly upset with the poor prognosis, and the situation begins to escalate. The patient's care team includes nurses, doctors, a social worker, and other ancillary staff. They must all remain calm, provide consistent messaging regarding the medical updates, and validate the family's emotions during this difficult time.

Practical Tips for De-escalating a Situation

Regis College [8] outlines ten essential tips for de-escalating a situation. These include:

- Maintaining nonthreatening body language.
- Standing approximately 3 feet away.
- Remaining calm and professional.
- Focusing on resolving the immediate issue.
- Demonstrating empathy.
- Allowing time for slow responses.
- Providing simple and clear instructions.

- Identifying the root cause of the problem.
- Being flexible when possible.
- Giving the individual time to process the situation.

With these tips in mind, healthcare providers can create a better environment for resolving conflict and improving patient outcomes.

Implementation Strategies

The Joint Commission describes three models of implementation strategies for de-escalation in the healthcare setting:

The Dix and Page model involves three components: assessment, communication, and tactics (ACT) [7]. This model emphasizes ongoing evaluation of the situation at hand and uses both verbal and nonverbal communication strategies that are tailored to the patient's present state [12]. It is an easy model for healthcare professionals to follow as it has a simple structure and promotes flexibility in choices based on real-time feedback [12].

The **Turnbull et al. model** is a feedback-based process that adjusts based on a patient's response during an escalating situation [7]. Key features of this model include ongoing monitoring of the aggressor's reaction and flexible and adaptable approaches that focus on the importance of understanding individual patient needs [7]. This model takes into consideration the fact that different interventions are effective for different people, so it is a highly individualized approach [7].

Finally, the **Safewards model** is a preventative and relationship-oriented framework. This model aims to prevent conflict and harm and is viewed as a holistic de-escalation process [12]. There are ten practical interventions in this model. Some of these include distraction tools, structured communication between patients and staff, and conflict avoidance techniques [7]. The Safewards model is evidence-based, resulting from a randomized controlled trial [7]. The emphasis is on a gradual process of enhancing patient and staff relationships and maintaining patient safety [7].

Techniques in Action

The following scenarios provide real-life examples of how de-escalation tactics can be successfully utilized in various healthcare-related situations. Each example highlights key strategies of de-escalation such as active listening, empathy, validation, and collaboration.

Scenario 1: A Patient with Poorly Managed Pain

A patient who feels her pain is not being well managed after a procedure may become irate and demand more medication. The healthcare professional might say, "I see you're in a lot of pain and I want to help. Let's talk about what we can do together to make you more comfortable." The provider's response validates the patient's feelings and invites the patient to collaborate on the next steps.

Scenario 2: A Family Member Who Is Upset

An angry father, upset with lack of updates on his daughter's condition, may may behave aggressively when the healthcare team approaches during rounds. The doctor might say in response, "I can understand your frustration and I can tell you are scared. Let me collect the most recent information and I will be back and share updated labs with you soon." This response is empathetic and provides a solution that can be acted on.

Scenario 3: A Patient Who Refuses Medical Treatment

When a patient refuses medical treatment and then becomes combative, a very simple statement about their autonomy can work wonders. The provider could state, "I realize you are uncomfortable with the proposed treatment. I respect your right to make decisions about your care. Let's talk more about your concerns so we can come to a solution that you are comfortable with." This strategy adheres to the principle of shared decision-making [13].

Outcomes of Using De-escalation Techniques in Healthcare

There are many advantages of using de-escalation techniques in healthcare settings. The Joint Commission [7] reports various positive outcomes according to some de-escalation studies. These include:

- Preventing violent behavior.
- Avoiding the use of restraint.
- Reducing anger and frustration.
- Maintaining the safety of staff and patients.
- Improving staff-patient connections.
- Enabling patients to manage their own emotions and regain personal control.
- Helping patients to develop feelings of hope, security, and self-acceptance.

Limitations

Surprisingly, there is no consensus on the best approach concerning de-escalation techniques. While there has been some research on this subject, there is limited research focusing on which techniques would be considered the "gold standard" [7]. This lack of standardization makes it challenging to measure long-term outcomes, particularly across various healthcare environments [10]. There is a need to conduct randomized controlled trials that compare de-escalation strategies, and the result would provide a much more robust evidence base around de-escalation techniques in healthcare [3].

Conclusion

The de-escalation techniques that are covered in this chapter are helpful tools in managing challenging patient and family interactions in the healthcare setting. These techniques can help to reduce tension and create a collaborative approach to care. Of course, challenges will remain, highlighting the need for more research and improved training in de-escalation techniques to help improve the overall healthcare experience for both patients and healthcare professionals alike.

Clinical Takeaways

Understanding the Root Causes of Difficult Behaviors

- Challenging patient interactions often stem from psychological, social, or systemic factors.
- Common contributors include anxiety, fear, communication barriers, past negative healthcare experiences, and mental health disorders.

Defining De-escalation

- De-escalation is a structured approach aimed at reducing patient agitation and preventing escalation of aggression.

Key De-escalation Strategies for Healthcare Professionals

- **Effective communication:** Use active listening, empathy, and calm verbal responses.
- **Nonverbal techniques:** Maintain an open posture, appropriate distance, and eye contact.

- **Environmental modifications:** Reduce noise, ensure privacy, and create a calm atmosphere.
- **Recognizing triggers and early signs:** Identify agitation signs early to intervene before escalation.
- **Collaboration among staff:** Ensure team consistency in messaging and approach with patients and families.

Implementation Models and Benefits

- Models like Dix and Page, Safewards, and Turnbull et al. emphasize structured de-escalation.
- Aims to reduce violent behavior, maintain safety of staff and patients, and improve patient-provider relationships.

Challenges and Areas for Improvement

- There is no standardized "gold standard" de-escalation technique.
- More research and training are needed to refine best practices and improve outcomes across different healthcare settings.

References

1. Iennaco J, Dixon J, Whittemore R, Bowers L. Measurement and monitoring of health care worker aggression exposure. Online J Issues Nurs. 2013;18(1) Manuscript 3. Available from: https://ojin.nursingworld.org/table-of-contents/volume-18-2013/number-1-january-2013/measurement-and-monitoring-worker-aggression-exposure/
2. Shenai N, Fulmer V, Gowl C, See J, Peterson R, Van Deusen R. A verbal de-escalation standardized patient workshop for third- and fourth-year medical students. MedEdPORTAL. 2024;20:11417. https://doi.org/10.15766/mep_2374-8265.11417.
3. Inglis P, Clifton A. De-escalation: the evidence, policy and practice. Journal of Intellectual Disabilities and Offending Behaviour. 2013;4(3):100–8.
4. Hardavella G, Aamli-Gaagnat A, Frille A, Saad N, Niculescu A, Powell P. Top tips to deal with challenging situations: doctor–patient interactions. Breathe (Sheff). 2017;13(2):129–35.
5. Jackson JL, Kay C, Scholcoff C, Becher D, O'Malley PG. Capturing the complexities of "difficult" patient encounters using a structural equation model. J Gen Intern Med. 2021;36(2):549–51. https://doi.org/10.1007/s11606-020-06013-8. Epub 2020 Jul 29. PMID:32728955;

PMCID:PMC7878594. Available from: https://pmc.ncbi.nlm.nih.gov/articles/PMC7878594/

6. Hahn SR, Kroenke K, Spitzer RL, Brody D, Williams JB, Linzer M, de Gruy FV 3rd. The difficult patient: prevalence, psychopathology, and functional impairment. J Gen Intern Med. 1996;11(1):1–8. https://doi.org/10.1007/BF02603477.
7. The Joint Commission. De-escalation in healthcare settings. The Joint Commission. 2018. Available from: https://www.jointcommission.org/-/media/tjc/newsletters/qs-47-deescalation-1-28-18-rev5.pdf
8. Regis College. De-escalation skills in mental health. Available from: https://online.regiscollege.edu/blog/de-escalation-skills-in-mental-health/
9. McKnight SE. De-escalating violence in healthcare: strategies to reduce emotional tension and aggression. 1st ed. Cham: Springer; 2020.
10. Price O, Baker J. Key components of de-escalation techniques: a thematic synthesis. Int J Ment Health Nurs. 2012;21(4):310–9. https://doi.org/10.1111/j.1447-0349.2011.00793.x.
11. Mulkey MA, Munro CL. Calming the agitated patient: providing strategies to support clinicians. Medsurg Nurs. 2021;30(1):9–13.
12. International Association for Healthcare Security and Safety Foundation. Mitigating workplace violence via de-escalation training. IAHSS Foundation; 2018 [cited 2024 Dec 27]. Available from: https://iahssf.org/assets/IAHSS-Foundation-De-Escalation-Training.pdf
13. Elwyn G, Frosch D, Thomson R, Joseph-Williams N, Lloyd A, Kinnersley P, et al. Shared decision making: a model for clinical practice. J Gen Intern Med. 2012;27(10):1361–7. https://doi.org/10.1007/s11606-012-2077-6.

9 Dismissal of Patient and Family from Practice

Yolanda Troublefield and Eileen Raynor

Dismissal of patients and families is typically seen as a "last resort." This is often after every effort has been made to ensure two-way communication, clear goals for care, mutual respect, and understanding. There are situations, however, where the patients' goals and provider care plan cannot be reconciled. Recently, the literature has seen an uptick in these situations regarding care for unvaccinated patients, particularly since the COVID-19 pandemic. Another area where this has been more common is in mental health patients where unaddressed mental health problems can exacerbate physical problems leading to mistrust and misunderstandings [1]. Focus on shared decision-making, careful explanation of the problem, and providing options for treatment work well for many patients; however, in the case of mental health conditions, this frequently fails to resolve concerns or improve treatment adherence. [1] Stivers et al. looked at patients presenting to clinics in the United Kingdom with depression symptoms and

Y. Troublefield
Private Practice, Dartmouth, MA, USA

E. Raynor (✉)
Head and Neck Surgery & Communication Sciences, Duke University Health, Durham, NC, USA
e-mail: eileen.raynor@duke.edu

E. Raynor (ed.), *Managing Challenging Patients and Families in Health Care Settings*, https://doi.org/10.1007/978-3-032-10492-2_9

found that refocusing the conversations around symptoms and the patients' perceptions as well as using the patients' own words was beneficial in helping overcome resistance to treatment even after several refusals. Here we can see how a strong patient-physician relationship can overcome obstacles including patient refusal of treatment options.

One concern is when patients fail to voice their desires or expectations. The physician-patient relationship depends on trust and honest transfer of information. Understanding the patient's expectations and formulating an appropriate response is fundamental to the shared decision-making model [2]. One study looked at this by surveying patients before and after treatment to find out what questions they may have had but did not articulate. A large number were based on interest in a second opinion, specialist referral, or more medical information [2]. Recognition of the "unspoken" by either asking the patient directly, identifying nonverbal cues, or allowing the patients some time to come back with questions may alleviate some of the anxiety related to unanswered expectations.

Physician characteristics associated with this concept of a strong physician-patient relationship include (1) a commitment to promote the health and well-being of patients, (2) a (qualified) willingness to subordinate one's own interests to the health interests of patients, and (3) a commitment to earn and maintain patient trust [3]. This is referred to the beneficence-fidelity model and is widely embraced by professional medical organizations. In cases where the physician has to terminate the relationship, they are obligated to notify the patient of their intent, have a satisfactory justification for this course of action, and provide sufficient opportunity to find another provider to take care of the patient. This is important to avoid patient abandonment which is widely prohibited [3]. Abandonment is defined by the AMA as:

> Physicians have an obligation to support continuity of care for their patients. While physicians have the option of withdrawing from a case, they cannot do so without giving notice to the patient, the relatives, or responsible friends sufficiently long in advance of withdrawal to permit another medical attendant to be secured [4].

Some justifications for "firing" patients have been proposed including the following: the patient lacks commitment to their personal health, futile utilization of healthcare resources and time, lack of accountability for one's health, and use as a tool to promote desirable changes in behavior by patients [3]. This logic is flawed on several levels, and studies have demonstrated that while patients may not be fully adherent to treatment plans, or have other reasons for refusal of treatment, i.e., vaccines, this does not mean they are not interested in being healthy or having health problems addressed. In situations where there may be a different provider that can effectively work with the patient and/or family, that may be a justifiable reason for termination of the relationship. Another case is when there is a risk that continuing the relationship is counterproductive or harmful to the patient.

Clinical Scenario

A 5 month old and his three siblings are all unvaccinated and present to their pediatrician office with 3 days of cough and worsening shortness of breath. The 5-month-old seems particularly more impacted, has noisy breathing, and is panting. There is a concern for possible epiglottis, and there are numerous children in the waiting area, some on steroids or immune modulators due to autoimmune conditions. The PCP wants to send the 5-month-old to the ED and is also concerned about possible infection of the other patients in the waiting room.

Issues for Potential Patient Harm

Having unimmunized patients in the office with possible sick or immunocompromised patients is a significant concern for many physicians. Numerous articles have been published recently due to an increasing number of pediatricians particularly dismissing unimmunized patients or families from their practices. [5–9] This has generated a large amount of controversy due to balancing the needs of the patient and the need of the community at large. One article mentioned the need for a written policy by the practice regarding patient dismissal, documentation of a conversation with the family regarding the risks to the patient and others of contracting a vaccine-preventable disease, addressing any concerns they have related to vaccinations, and parent responsibility to inform providers of the immunization status [6, 10]. The American Academy of Pediatrics has provided a "refusal to vaccinate" form that can be given to parents. Another study looked at the impact of "zero tolerance" vaccine policy and found more clustering of unvaccinated patients into fewer practices with problems regarding access for care as well as lower likelihood of developing any herd immunity. The study concluded that the risk of transmission of disease in a diverse practice is much less than the impact of clustering unimmunized patients into fewer, more tolerant practices [7]. An editorial described this as a "slippery slope" questioning other areas where patients may not follow recommendations and then be dismissed from the practice [8]. In some cases, dismissal of a family from the practice due to not vaccinating can be viewed as a form of coercion; however, there is not data showing this action actually changed someone's decision whether or not to vaccinate their child [10]. In states with more lenient exemption policies, this study showed more practices dismissing unvaccinated patients. This was also more evident in the Southern United States and in suburban settings [10].

Legal Considerations

Clear and consistent documentation is vital to demonstrate that a good faith effort was made to inform patients of decision to terminate the relationship. One recommendation is to send two letters, one via routine mail and a follow-up by registered mail requiring an acceptance signature for the document. Ensuring correct contact information at each patient visit is key to making sure accuracy and avoidance of returned mail. Clinical documentation of treatment plans, risks if not followed, and follow-up recommendations are also important to prevent potential for liability claim once a patient is dismissed from the practice [11]. There are several clear/straightforward situations where it is reasonable to consider termination of the relationship. These include drug-seeking behaviors, violence or threats to the medical staff, falsification of records, or theft [12]. Knowing state laws and state medical licensing board rules regarding these conditions and best way to document is imperative to prevent legal recourse from the patient.

Summary

Releasing patients from medical practices can have significant medical and legal implications for the patient and for the provider. This "nuclear" option should be reserved only when all other means of communication have failed or in cases of threatened harm to staff or the facility.

Clinical Pearls

- Know state laws and state medical board rules on abandonment, dismissal, and options for mitigation.
- Consider working with someone else in the practice to be able to preserve the patient relationship and care.
- Have a plan for referral should the patient need to be dismissed and make sure that is well documented.
- Document everything clearly so there is no difficulty in understanding why the patient or family were "fired."
- Consider mental health issues and referral if that is part of the challenge with managing the patients' condition.

References

1. Stivers T, McCabe R. Dueling in the clinic: when patients and providers disagree about healthcare recommendations. Soc Sci Med. 2021;290:114140.
2. Bell RA, Kravitz RL, Thom D, Krupat E, Azari R. Unsaid but not forgotten: patients' unvoiced desires in office visits. Arch Intern Med. 2001;161(16):1977–84. https://jamanetwork.com/journals/jamainternalmedicine/fullarticle/648933
3. Wicclair M. Dismissing patients for health-based reasons. Camb Q Healthc Ethics. 2013;22(3):308–18. https://www.cambridge.org/core/journals/cambridge-quarterly-of-healthcare-ethics/article/abs/

dismissing-patients-for-healthbased-reasons/39BBC05A88BB148E1145 16FAA9975054

4. Kuczewski MG. Brubaker L. AMA J Ethics. 2017;
5. MacDonald NE, Harmon S, Dube E, et al. Is physician dismissal of vaccine refusers an acceptable practice in Canada? A 2018 overview. Paediatr Child Health. 2019;24(2):92–7.
6. Brous E. Legal issues in dismissing unvaccinated patients. Am J Nurs. 2018;118(6):64–6.
7. Buttenheim AM, Cherng ST, Asch DA. Provider dismissal policies and clustering of vaccine-hesitant families: an agent-based modeling approach. Hum Vaccin Immunother. 2013;9(8):1819–24.
8. Elston MP. Dismissing families: a critical issue. Arch Pediatr Adolesc Med. 2006;160(4):452–3.
9. Flanagan-Klygis EA, Sharp L, Frader JE. Dismissing the family who refuses vaccines: a study of pediatrician attitudes. Arch Pediatr Adolesc Med. 2005;159(10):929–34.
10. Garcia TB, O'Leary ST. Dismissal policies for vaccine refusal among US physicians: a literature review. Hum Vaccin Immunother. 2020;16(5):1189–93.
11. Staff TRM. RM Matters/second chances: accepting a dismissed patient back into your practice. J Calif Dent Assoc. 2017;45(1):43–4.
12. Lippman H, Davenport J. Patient dismissal: the right way to do it. J Fam Pract. 2011;60(3)

10 Recognizing Your Own Emotional State

Chelsea Walsh

Exploring the Emotional Landscape

There are strategies to keep in mind for when your own emotions may be contributing to your assessment, communication, and plan for a patient. First, ask yourself: what emotion(s) am I feeling? Consider these examples:

- You may be feeling frustrated that the patient does not want to move forward with surgery when it is clearly beneficial.
- You may feel anxious because the patient's twin passed away in utero, and now the family presents for the first well-child check that should have been with two babies.
- You are discouraged that a patient's visiting family refuses to wear a mask on the oncology unit and it is flu season.
- A patient's insurance company denied coverage for a life-changing medication and you are exasperated.
- A situation has escalated to the point of dismissing a patient from practice, and you are feeling guilty yet angry.

C. Walsh (✉)
Duke Children's Hospital and Health Center, Durham, NC, USA
e-mail: Chelsea.walsh@duke.edu

E. Raynor (ed.), *Managing Challenging Patients and Families in Health Care Settings*, https://doi.org/10.1007/978-3-032-10492-2_10

These situations take a toll on healthcare professionals who care deeply about their patients and want to provide the best care. When "the best" is not achievable, it can create feelings of failure. Whatever may be the reason leading to a strong response, it is important to first identify the emotion.

Once the emotion is identified, one can then reflect on what factors led to this point. From the start, a challenging situation can cause tension and strong emotions. In contrast, sometimes the situation has been escalating over an extended amount of time. For example:

- You have been communicating with the patient's family for months about the same issue, without resolution.
- You have been on call for the past 48 hours and are exhausted, both physically and mentally, but a patient's family is requesting you at bedside with concerns of the care their loved one has received.
- For the past 6 months, your clinic has been understaffed with a huge caseload and little room to breathe, and now a patient is concerned that you have not responded to their healthcare portal message in 3 days.

Both the patient and your concerns are valid, and sometimes we do not have control over any of the results or necessary next steps. What we can work to control are our emotional responses to events and situations such as those presented above.

Sympathy Versus Empathy

Clinical Scenario

William, a 62-year-old male, underwent a liver transplant yesterday. He is in pain and feels like his nurse is not keeping up with his scheduled pain regimen. He does not have any family with him at bedside and is unable to reach his call light. The next time his nurse enters the room he is very curt, mumbling under his breath that he needed help "since over an hour ago." The nurse apologizes, obtains a pain score, administers his pain medications, and then leaves quickly. She labels him as a grouch during report to the oncoming shift.

How could this situation have been handled differently? The nurse could have empathized with the patient and realized he was alone during a painful, frightening time in his life. His reaction, while not the most polite, is certainly a normal human response to a stressful situation.

An important emotional management skill in healthcare is learning to *empathize,* not sympathize. The definition of sympathy is "the act or capacity of entering into or sharing the feelings or interests of another" according to Merriam-Webster [1]. A small study of adult inpatient cancer patients demonstrated a preference toward the healthcare workers who exhibited compassion and empathy rather than sympathy [2]. Some patients described sympathy as an act of pity, and this was not well received from a patient standpoint. In comparison, the definition of empathy is "the action of understanding, being aware of, being sensitive to, and vicariously experiencing the feelings, thoughts, and experience of another" [3]. This is in line with the old phrase, "put yourself in their shoes." The healthcare members that provided empathy and compassion were much more personable and seemed to genuinely care for and understand what the patient was feeling [2].

However, there is a fine line between understanding and over-empathizing. In healthcare, it is important to recognize our empath etic thoughts are in response to something happening to someone else [4]. The events provoking empathetic thoughts are not occurring to the healthcare provider themselves, and it is essential that the provider is able to set and keep this boundary. This concept is known as the self-other distinction; if the self-other distinction becomes blurred, it can lead to compassion fatigue and burnout [4].

Consider this scenario: a child is placed in foster care, and you feel connected because you went through the foster system as a child as well. This connection causes you to feel more deeply for this patient, and you decide to provide your personal cell phone number. This would be distorting the self-other distinction because your experience is not theirs and your emotions in the situation have caused a breach of boundaries. Over time, if one continued along this avenue for every foster child they met, they could become burned out, affecting care for themselves and everyone else.

Burnout and Compassion Fatigue

Clinical Scenario

Judy is a pediatrician who often overextends herself due to the deep desire of keeping patients and their families happy. A patient arrived 1 hour late for their appointment, and initially Judy said they would have to reschedule. The front desk calls back a few minutes later to say that the patient's parent is irate and demands to be seen, touting traffic as the reason for tardiness. Judy acquiesces even though it causes her to be late for her own child's soccer game. Over the next several years, Judy continues to accommodate requests at the expense of her own private life and eventually becomes burned out. She leaves primary care for the research sector.

Burnout in healthcare is an extremely common issue and contributes to emotional well-being, too. According to the World Health Organization's ICD-11, "Burnout is a syndrome conceptualized as resulting from chronic workplace stress that has not been successfully managed" [5]. Burnout is further characterized into three subgroups described as emotional exhaustion, depersonalization, and the loss of personal accomplishment [5].

During the Covid-19 pandemic, burnout rates skyrocketed. A study of healthcare professionals including dieticians, nurses, physicians, occupational therapists, and respiratory therapists found there was a statistically significant difference in relative hair cortisol levels collected throughout the pandemic that was associated with burnout symptoms among the participants. The highest proportions of burnout were measured in Quarter 1 (57.3%) and Quarter 3 (59.6%) of the pandemic [6]. Factors that may lead to burnout include, "heavy workload, high job demands, inadequate skills, difficult work conditions, lack of supportive supervision, low career satisfaction, poor wages, job insecurity, fewer qualifications, less experience, exposure to workplace violence, and low social support" [7].

Anecdotally, healthcare systems and private practices are often striving to fit as many patients in a workday as possible whether it is for profit, patient satisfaction, or other driving forces. This leads to double- or triple-booking providers in the name of providing good, timely patient care. But what does this do to our mental health and emotional state? Often, rushed days may lead to physical and mental fatigue, inaccurate decision-making, and poor patient satisfaction. And, in an already challenging patient, a rushed visit or conversation can lead to more frustration with both parties if neither feels the needs are adequately being met.

Unconscious Bias

Clinical Scenario

In a labor and delivery ward, a baby is born with features characteristic of fetal alcohol syndrome. Multiple members of the care team during rounds quickly begin discussing how it is selfish of the mom to drink alcohol without caring about what it does to her infant. They gawk at the fact that she did not receive any prenatal care, either. Later they learn she was a victim of sex trafficking which caused her to become pregnant, and she used alcohol to cope with this trauma.

This scenario depicts implicit bias as the care team instinctively assumed the mother was selfish due to baby having fetal alcohol syndrome. Implicit bias is dangerous as it can lead to clouded decision-making.

Whether one wants to acknowledge or not, we all exhibit implicit, or unconscious, bias. This bias is not readily recognized by individuals and could be a bias toward race, ethnicity, LGBTQ status, sex, weight, or religious beliefs, for example [8]. The extent to which unconscious bias affects clinical decision-making is still being studied, but due to the nature of implicit bias being "unconscious," we are not readily aware of the bias occurring in the moment. Strategies to counter unconscious bias include education academically and institutionally, along with self-reflection [8]. Medical school and allied healthcare programs can provide courses to address these biases and techniques to become more self-aware. Larger healthcare systems may consider annual implicit bias refreshers.

Resilience

Recognizing your own emotional state is important not only in the workplace but at home too. The timeless adage, "take care of yourself or you cannot take care of others," remains relevant. Ensuring you have plenty of rest, good nutrition, exercise, and relaxation are all essential basics to maintaining good health physically and mentally. Stress, anxiety, and fatigue may take a toll on your day-to-day emotional well-being, and finding a healthy coping mechanism(s) to manage these symptoms and emotions is essential. Some relate good coping with resilience. Resilience was previously thought to be tied to personality traits, but in the past decade, resilience was found to be a characteristic that can be learned [9]. Due to this shift in thought around fostering resilience, many medical and allied health programs are beginning to educate students about the importance of resilience so they may grow in their careers successfully while maintaining a positive attitude [7].

Nurturing resilience is an excellent way to stay energized, focused, and successful in a workplace setting that can sometimes be chaotic or challenging. With the right tools in your toolbelt, you can be successful during and after difficult situations to maintain a positive emotional state and reaction.

Working in the field of healthcare is extremely rewarding but can be taxing due to the intrinsic nature of caring for those with illnesses. By periodically reflecting on your own emotional awareness and mental health, and with the proper resiliency training, you can remain successful in sharing your expertise while keeping a positive outlook, even in the most difficult of situations.

Key Takeaways

- Healthcare workers should try to embody empathy rather than sympathy with patients.
- Recognizing burnout and compassion fatigue will allow for better responses to challenging patient situations.
- Everyone has implicit bias—what one does with this knowledge can help them manage difficult situations in a professional manner.
- Resilience can be learned and nurtured with coping strategies and early education.

References

1. America's most trusted dictionary. In: Merriam-Webster. https://www.merriam-webster.com/dictionary/sympathy. Accessed 19 Nov 2024.
2. Sinclair S, Beamer K, Hack TF, McClement S, Raffin Bouchal S, Chochinov HM, Hagen NA. Sympathy, empathy, and compassion: a grounded theory study of palliative care patients' understandings, experiences, and preferences. Palliat Med. 2016;31:437–47.
3. America's most trusted dictionary. In: Merriam-Webster. https://www.merriam-webster.com/dictionary/empathy. Accessed 19 Nov 2024.
4. Hofmeyer A, Taylor R, Kennedy K. Knowledge for nurses to better care for themselves so they can better care for others during the COVID-19 pandemic and beyond. Nurse Educ Today. 2020;94:104503.
5. Burn-out an "Occupational phenomenon": International Classification of Diseases. In: World Health Organization. https://www.who.int/news/item/28-05-2019-burn-out-an-occupational-phenomenon-international-classification-of-diseases. Accessed 14 Nov 2024.
6. Marcil M-J, Cyr S, Marin M-F, et al. Hair cortisol change at covid-19 pandemic onset predicts burnout among health personnel. Psychoneuroendocrinology. 2022;138:105645.
7. Thapa DK, Levett-Jones T, West S, Cleary M. Burnout, compassion fatigue, and resilience among healthcare professionals. Nurs Health Sci. 2021;23:565–9.
8. Marcelin JR, Siraj DS, Victor R, Kotadia S, Maldonado YA. The impact of unconscious bias in healthcare: how to recognize and mitigate it. J Infect Dis. 2019; https://doi.org/10.1093/infdis/jiz214.
9. Chmitorz A, Kunzler A, Helmreich I, Tüscher O, Kalisch R, Kubiak T, Wessa M, Lieb K. Intervention studies to foster resilience—a systematic review and proposal for a resilience framework in future intervention studies. Clin Psychol Rev. 2018;59:78–100.

When to Call in Reinforcements

11

Eileen Raynor

Difficulty Communicating with the Patient

Clinical Scenario **A 7-year-old with Spanish-speaking parents seeking treatment for sleep-disordered breathing and large tonsils. Family recent immigrants from Central America. Have concerns that taking out tonsils causes sterility. Video interpreter only is available.**

Communication is critical to understanding what the patient is being seen for, what the problem is, and mitigating or historical factors that may impact the diagnoses and conveying next steps. In earlier chapters, we discussed issues such as language barriers and health literacy. Determining where the patient or family member speaking for the patient is in terms of emotional state, ability to speak clearly, and ability to convey information and appropriately answer questions, primary language and how "literate" they are regarding their health is vital to establishing a beneficial professional healthcare relationship. In the simplest of cases, the problem is language discordance between the patient/family and

E. Raynor (✉)
Head and Neck Surgery & Communication Sciences, Duke University Health, Durham, NC, USA
e-mail: eileen.raynor@duke.edu

E. Raynor (ed.), *Managing Challenging Patients and Families in Health Care Settings*, https://doi.org/10.1007/978-3-032-10492-2_11

healthcare provider, and the reinforcement needed is a medical interpreter who is able to transfer information reliably between the different languages. Multiple studies have shown increased emergency department (ED) utilization when the use of interpreters is not available [1]. Adult and pediatric patients impacted by language-related barriers are especially vulnerable during care transitions, especially with transitions from the hospital or ED to home. Up to 27% of language discordant people experienced an adverse event within the 2 weeks after discharge [2].

In other cases, this may be more complicated, such as when the patient or family member interrupts the discussion with unrelated comments or questions, or one or more of the party get upset with the information being discussed. At such times, it may be beneficial to “take 5” and give them a few minutes to themselves to settle down, reframe the discussion, and then proceed. Asking another staff member to be present in the exam room is a way to provide some extra support for the physician and the patient or family member who is having an emotional reaction or being disruptive to the medical encounter. In some situations, the family member may be asked to step out of the room in order to gather the necessary information from the patient.

In cases when young children are accompanying the patient, it can be helpful to ask a medical staff assistant or child life specialist to help distract the other family members so parents or the patient can focus on what is happening. In the age of electronics and social media, it is not uncommon for the patient or others to be using their tablet or phone during the encounter which creates a significant distraction to the patient and provider conversation. In those cases, asking them to please complete their business after the visit so they can have your (and you their) undivided attention will establish an environment to provide the best medical decision-making allowable. Ensuring a direct line of communication with attentiveness to the discussion is imperative to ensure the best possible outcome regarding medical decision-making and treatment. Maintaining a professional demeanor and keeping eye contact and an attentive posture will typically cause the patient to mirror those actions and therefore allow for more effective transfer of information [3].

Sometimes the information being discussed is quite distressing, and it can be helpful for the patient to have another family member or close friend present for the visit to be a support, ask questions, and take notes for the patient [4]. If there is not someone present during the clinic visit for the patient, giving them an opportunity to either call someone or plan a follow-up so they can have their support person can make a big difference to their emotional well-being. Additionally, physicians are not always good at detecting patient distress during bad news encounters, which may negatively affect patient experience. Feedback from an independent observer has been demonstrated to improve physician self-perception of their communication skill, especially in emotionally charged situations [4]. Effective communication between healthcare providers and accompanying persons can help ease anxiety and improve patient outcomes [5].

The principal foundation in each of these situations is establishment of trust. The use of patient-centered communication and taking time to sit, make eye contact, and actively listen are important steps the healthcare provider can take to establish a caring environment that lends itself to creating a safe space for the patient interaction [6, 7]. In the context of patient–physician relationships, patient-centered communication is particularly important to mitigate patient–provider conflicts since this may include exchanging information and responding to emotions, thus helping patients manage uncertainty and make good decisions about their health [8, 9]. Patient-centered communication has the potential to reduce patients' illness uncertainty, medical setting uncertainty, and relational uncertainty and to promote a better understanding of their doctors' motivation [8]. Thom and Campbell found that if doctors convey to their patients that they understand a patient's health concerns, illness, and emotional status and express their concern and care for the patient and his or her well-being, patient trust will increase [6, 10]. The uncertainty of illness and complexity of diagnostic practices have contributed to the increasingly strained relationship, which can impede healthcare provision and patient outcomes. Thus, there is a significant need to establish and maintain a mutually trusting and beneficial relationship between doctors and patients [8].

Difficulty Communicating with the Caregiver

Clinical Scenario A 21-year-old with Down syndrome presents to the ED with signs of appendicitis accompanied by a friend from a group home.

In many instances, the patient is accompanied by a caregiver such as a parent, guardian, or adult children. Most of the time these extra people are there specifically for the patient's well-being; however, at times there may be disagreement between the patient and family member on how to proceed with the medical recommendations. This is quite apparent in elder care when adult children may not agree with the patient's living will or care wishes. A living will places the right to refuse lifesaving treatment into the context of informed consent [11]. In those cases, having a case manager or social worker speak with the patient and family separately can be useful, especially if the patient is cognitively able to make their own healthcare decisions. In most states, guardians are charged by statute with exercising "substituted judgment" for or acting in the "best interests of" the wards in their charge [11]. Guardians serve principally as alter egos of the ward with regard to personal decision-making; they have both the authority and the obligation to assure that the ward's legal right to autonomy in medical decision-making is respected and enforced [11, 12]. The concept of "healthcare power of attorney" became popularized after its introduction into California statute, ensuring that "an individual can legally designate a surrogate to make healthcare decisions when the individual becomes incapacitated." [11] Several rulings by the courts have determined that a court-appointed guardian is obligated to ensure that the ward's own preferences are reflected in every healthcare-related decision the guardian makes, in every context, unless doing so is impossible [11, 12]. This is in keeping with the concept that the individual is allowed "personal liberty" when medical treatment is involved. Encouraging patients to set up living wills and healthcare power of attorneys while they still have capacity to identify these persons and clearly define their wishes is an important aspect to ensuring fewer conflicts should this situation arise [12].

Other times there may be joint custody issues in the care of a minor where the parents do not agree on what to do for the child. In cases of sexual health, this is even more sensitive, and expectations of the patient and parents may be quite divergent [13, 14]. Utilizing other resources such as the patient's primary care or providing clear information to the family on the recommendations and rationale behind them (unless in an emergency situation) and allowing them time to think separately and return at another time to decide on next steps may be the best way to allow parents to make a decision they can agree on. Encouraging obtaining a second opinion where appropriate is another tool that can help families come to a mutually agreed-upon decision. One study examined frequent primary care attenders and the use of a multidisciplinary referral clinic. They found this met the needs of the patient and provider as well as lowering costs for medical care. Employing a model like this for patients where there are differences in opinion regarding management or persistent concern about symptoms that are nonorganic in nature may be an option to help the patient achieve their goals in a cost-effective yet satisfactory manner [15].

The use of online health resources has become much more prevalent over recent years, and these resources may be driving some of the patient or family medical decision-making. In some cases, the use of online health communities, especially when dealing with chronic conditions, can actually serve as a support and provide health-related information that has been vetted for accuracy. The utilization of these external sources in many cases improved adherence to the medical treatment plan [9]. The patient portal, another venue used by patients to ask questions from the healthcare team, is another method that seems to improve overall communication and patient satisfaction of their care. A different chapter takes a deeper look into custody issues that arise within the healthcare environment and how to ensure compliance with these laws.

Adolescence is a particularly difficult time with regard to privacy versus autonomy for the patient. In several studies, parents agreed that confidential care may increase adolescent comfort and honesty when talking to providers about health concerns, yet many parents desired full disclosure of information from the physician once the information was shared with the patient [16]. When the patient is an adolescent discussing sensitive medical information, it may be useful to have the parents step out of the room and speak to the patient directly and then have another party, such as a nurse or medical assistant present when parents return to keep the discussion from becoming emotionally charged. Trust between adolescents and their healthcare providers is important for patient–provider rapport, an adolescent's developing autonomy, and providing a safe environment for disclosure of sensitive health concerns [16]. The assurance of confidentiality has been shown to increase an adolescent's willingness to disclose information about sexuality, substance use, and mental health and increase their intention to return to that same provider for future health concerns [14].

Threatening Situations

Workplace violence in healthcare settings has been escalating in recent years, particularly in emergency settings. Up to 12% of assaults in the USA occur in a healthcare setting, and in 20% of emergency departments (ED), guns or knives have been brought onto the premises [17]. Physician trainees are generally more vulnerable due to their relative inexperience and are usually less likely to report threatening situations [17, 18].

Many healthcare centers have started screening at the entrances to prevent firearms from being brought on-site. Most healthcare facilities have police or security available to intervene in a physically threatening situation; however, only a small percentage of them may actually be armed [18]. Smaller medical practices may not have this recourse and have to rely on 911 to respond if there is an active threat against a patient or medical staff. States have enacted legislation aimed at reducing violence in healthcare settings, but these are not often as much of a deterrent as would be preferred. If one is found to be in a situation where there is a threat made, the first step is isolating the person from others, calling for help, and keeping the person calm as much as possible. Many of the patients or accompanying persons are under the influence of alcohol or other illicit substances or having a mental health crisis that is driving the aggressive behavior. One study used survey data and a workshop to help ED staff mitigate these situations, and while they did not find a reduction in violent threats overall, they did find the respondents felt safer overall with more event reporting and documentation of the events [19]. Still, there is a significant lack of training for dealing with these situations. One survey of emergency room physicians found that they desired training in de-escalation techniques, conflict management, and identification of threats [18].

Critical to de-escalation, strong interpersonal communication is crucial for individuals coping with threats in the workplace, especially for hospitals that provide high-quality care and patient safety [5]. Involving a multiprofessional team and security measures are ways that some of these threats may be managed in a safe way for staff and patients. Role-playing and scenarios or simulations are also useful tools to practice these measures such that the actions required become more ingrained.

Inability to Come to a Reasonable Conclusion on Treatment

Clinical Scenario A 10-year-old with confirmed acute strep throat. Parent insists on "homeopathic" treatment, does not "trust medicines," and gets visibly upset when told the child really needs antibiotics due to the risks of untreated strep infection.

The use of complementary and alternative medicine has risen over the last decade. These therapies include herbal supplements, Chinese medicine, chiropractor manipulation, and the use of vitamins or minerals for a variety of health conditions [20]. It is estimated the anywhere from 20% to 45% of pediatric patients in the USA have used some form of homeopathic remedies. Many parents or patients do not disclose the use of these treatments to their provider fearing shaming, or they feel these are completely safe since they do not require a prescription. Most of these do not undergo the vigors of clinical trials yet can have significant health impacts, especially if combined with some prescription medications [20]. Having open, candid discussion with parents and patients about the risks and possible benefits of these therapies and, when possible, keeping a balanced approach while counseling on what to watch for is a reasonable way to mitigate use of these substances. Avoiding introduction of attitudes and biases will also encourage open communication by the parent and patient on what they are actually taking for their condition aside from that medically recommended [3].

Sometimes, despite all our best efforts, there is disagreement on how to proceed with care management or treatment by the patient, family, and healthcare provider. In those cases, arranging for a second opinion and providing other resources can allow time for education and discussion. Printed or vetted online materials can be useful to help with patient education regarding treatment options and give the patient a chance to process what was presented to them. Instances where there is dissatisfaction with the provider–patient relationship were typically related to areas of communication. Insufficient information, insufficient respect, and insufficient empathy were described as the most common reasons for a negative professional encounter [21].

Intercultural differences also play a significant role in these types of situations. One finds that in multicultural societies, there are challenges for health communication related to a lack of shared meaning and differences in language and cultural practices [13]. This creates issues with misunderstandings and can hinder the underlying trust that the patient places on the physician. "Truth telling" and having an empathetic, straightforward, and ethical discussion around the diagnosis and treatment should be emphasized [13].

Gender segregation due to religious beliefs and cultural traditions also present intercultural communication challenges between patients and health professionals. Female patients from cultures with gender segregation often report feeling uncomfortable to be seen by male doctors or nurses. This could lead to patients refusing to turn up for scheduled appointments, to the delay of treatments, and to the waste of medical resources [13].

Ensuring these patients have access to gender-friendly care, respecting their privacy wishes, and keeping the communication open are methods that can ensure the patients get the appropriate care needed.

Unclear Who Is Actually the "Legal Guardian"

Clinical Scenario A 3-year-old accompanied by adult sister, aunt, and grandmother for severe asthma exacerbation and needs hospital admission.

Children are typically brought to the healthcare provider by their parent or legal guardian, but there are often times where the person bringing the child in is not their guardian. Sometimes these are relatives of the child or parent, but they may also be a sibling or family friend. These persons may not self-identify unless directly asked how they are related to the patient. It is important to identify the relationship of the accompanying person, and if they are not the parent or legal guardian, attempts must be made to speak with the legal guardian prior to initiation of the medical encounter. The parent may be reachable by telephone and give verbal consent for the child to be seen and cared for, or they may provide a signed note to that effect.

When the child is in foster care, there are specific situations that the foster parent can consent to such as evaluation and treatment but not invasive procedure. If there is any question about the legality of the guardian, especially in adoption cases, paperwork should be obtained and on file in the system for future reference. A clinical social worker can confirm this as well. Contacting the DSS case worker may be necessary to determine who is legally allowed to consent for care and treatment of the patient. The informed consent is a legal document whose use has been expanded to include surgery, medical treatments, and research. It is defined as the "right of a competent patient to unwanted medical treatment even in cases where this may be lifesaving." [11] There are specific exceptions in emergency situations where the patient cannot consent for themselves and there is not enough time to find a legal representative to sign for the patient. This definition includes (1) an immediate, clear threat to life or limb; (2) treatment must be in line with the standard of care for the condition; and (3) time needed to obtain informed consent would drastically increase risk of morbidity or mortality (such as acute hemorrhage or airway obstruction) [11].

Summary

The underlying link in all these situations is effective communication. This may necessitate the use of other individuals to help either mitigate and provide support for an emotional encounter, provide interpreter services for language disparities, clarify cultural differences, or ensure a safe alternative space for accompanying family members, so the patient is free to communicate with their healthcare provider. The establishment of trust is paramount to ensuring the patient and caregivers are able to understand the medical condition, ask pertinent questions, and be actively involved in any medical decision-making such as treatment options. When communication becomes inhibited, the use of additional personnel, providing resources, or offering a second opinion may still preserve the physician–patient relationship and allow for the desired health outcomes.

Clinical Takeaways

- Keeping in mind communication is critical to transfer of information and ensuring best possible care, identify what steps are needed to ensure that communication is possible.
- Utilization of members of the healthcare team can help with keeping family members from distracting the patient and provider interaction.
- Case managers and clinical social workers are valuable in determining legality of guardianship and medical decision-making.
- Offering a break "take 5" and providing resources may help families and patients absorb upsetting/disturbing medical information and allow for continuation of the conversation.

– Offering a second opinion or the use of a care navigator in cases where appropriate may help patients/families come to a decision when they do not agree with recommendations.

References

1. Chu JN, Wong J, Bardach NS, et al. Association between language discordance and unplanned hospital readmissions or emergency department revisits: a systematic review and meta-analysis. BMJ Qual Saf. 2024;33(7):456–69. In eng. https://doi.org/10.1136/bmjqs-2023-016295.
2. Forster AJ, Murff HJ, Peterson JF, Gandhi TK, Bates DW. The incidence and severity of adverse events affecting patients after discharge from the hospital. Ann Intern Med. 2003;138(3):161–7. In eng. https://doi.org/10.7326/0003-4819-138-3-200302040-00007.
3. Chichirez C-M, Purcărea V. Interpersonal communication in healthcare. J Med Life. 2018;11(2):119.
4. Lee SJ, Back AL, Block SD, Stewart SK. Enhancing physician-patient communication. ASH Educ Program Book. 2002;2002(1):464–83.
5. Dietl JE, Derksen C, Keller FM, Schmiedhofer M, Lippke S. psychosocial processes in healthcare workers: how individuals' perceptions of interpersonal communication is related to patient safety threats and higher-quality care. Int J Environ Res Public Health. 2023;20(9):5698.
6. Lee YY, Lin JL. Linking patients' trust in physicians to health outcomes Br J Hosp Med (Lond). 2008;69(1):42–6. In eng. https://doi.org/10.12968/hmed.2008.69.1.28040.
7. Mast MS. On the importance of nonverbal communication in the physician–patient interaction. Patient Educ Couns. 2007;67(3):315–8.
8. Chen L, Tang H, Guo Y. Effect of patient-centered communication on physician-patient conflicts from the physicians' perspective: a moderated mediation model. J Health Commun. 2022;27(3):164–72.
9. Lu X, Zhang R. Impact of physician-patient communication in online health communities on patient compliance: cross-sectional questionnaire study. J Med Internet Res. 2019;21(5):e12891. In eng. https://doi.org/10.2196/12891.
10. Thom DH, Campbell B. Patient-physician trust: an exploratory study. J Fam Pract. 1997;44(2):169–76. In eng
11. Dayton K. Standards for health care decision-making: legal and practical considerations. Utah L Rev. 2012:1329.
12. Zietlow K, Dubin L, Battles A, Vitale C. Guardianship: a medicolegal review for clinicians. J Am Geriatr Soc. 2022;70(11):3070–9.
13. Zhao X. Challenges and barriers in intercultural communication between patients with immigration backgrounds and health professionals: a sys-

tematic literature review. Health Commun. 2023;38(4):824–33. https://doi.org/10.1080/10410236.2021.1980188.
14. Ford CA, Millstein SG, Halpern-Felsher BL, Irwin CE Jr. Influence of physician confidentiality assurances on adolescents' willingness to disclose information and seek future health care: a randomized controlled trial. JAMA. 1997;278(12):1029–34. https://doi.org/10.1001/jama.1997.03550120089044.
15. Matalon A, Nahmani T, Rabin S, Maoz B, Hart J. A short-term intervention in a multidisciplinary referral clinic for primary care frequent attenders: description of the model, patient characteristics and their use of medical resources. Fam Pract. 2002;19(3):251–6. (In eng. https://doi.org/10.1093/fampra/19.3.251.
16. Bogart AR, Richards M, Sheeder J. Youth and guardian expectations of privacy in adolescent health care. J Adolesc Health. 2024;75(5):737–42.
17. Schnapp BH, Slovis BH, Shah AD, et al. Workplace violence and harassment against emergency medicine residents. West J Emerg Med. 2016;17(5):567–73. In eng. https://doi.org/10.5811/westjem.2016.6.30446.
18. Kowalenko T, Walters BL, Khare RK, Compton S. Workplace violence: a survey of emergency physicians in the state of Michigan. Ann Emerg Med. 2005;46(2):142–7. In eng. https://doi.org/10.1016/j.annemergmed.2004.10.010.
19. Fernandes CM, Raboud JM, Christenson JM, et al. The effect of an education program on violence in the emergency department. Ann Emerg Med. 2002;39(1):47–55. In eng. https://doi.org/10.1067/mem.2002.121202.
20. Children and natural health products: what a clinician should know. Paediatr Child Health. 2005;10(4):227–32. In eng. https://doi.org/10.1093/pch/10.4.227.
21. Jangland E, Gunningberg L, Carlsson M. Patients' and relatives' complaints about encounters and communication in health care: Evidence for quality improvement. Patient Educ Couns. 2009;75(2):199–204. https://doi.org/10.1016/j.pec.2008.10.007.

12 Wrap-Up and Summary

Eileen Raynor

Effective communication is the foundation of success in both personal and professional lives. It enables individuals to express their thoughts clearly, understand others, build strong relationships, and resolve conflicts efficiently. In healthcare, it is critical that communication be clear, bidirectional, and honest. This ensures the best possible outcomes for patients and maintains trust that is critical to the relationship.

Enhancing Relationships

Good communication fosters trust, understanding, and emotional connection. Active listening and open body language go a long way to provide the safe space needed to ensure the parties are all engaged in the discussion. Asking questions based on the responses heard, reframing the salient points, and summarizing at the end are useful ways to ensure that what was conveyed is the same as that received. Since the patient-provider relationship is

E. Raynor (✉)
Head and Neck Surgery & Communication Sciences, Duke University Health, Durham, NC, USA
e-mail: eileen.raynor@duke.edu

E. Raynor (ed.), *Managing Challenging Patients and Families in Health Care Settings*, https://doi.org/10.1007/978-3-032-10492-2_12

the most important aspect of the healthcare process, recognizing where there may be barriers to understanding or relating important information allows for a reset of the conversation and provides a path to move forward. This is dependent on figuring out where the patient's health literacy is, any language or cultural barriers, and identifying topics that are more uncomfortable so they can be approached in a caring and informed manner.

Increased Productivity and Efficiency

In a professional setting, clear communication ensures that tasks are understood and executed correctly. Miscommunication can lead to errors, delays, and frustration. Leaders who communicate well inspire and motivate their teams, leading to improved performance. As we discussed earlier in this book, use of teams, multiple methods of providing health information and ensuring that patients and families actually understand what and why certain recommendations are made are great methods for enhancing provider-patient communication. For teaching institutions, modeling this behavior and explicitly discussing the impact of communication on patients and families can help students and residents become more adept at working within interprofessional teams, teaching patients and families about their care plan, and understanding when there may need to be some other interventions or a third party to help if situations become too emotionally charged.

Preventing and Resolving Conflicts

Many conflicts arise due to misunderstandings. Effective communication helps in addressing issues openly, finding common ground, and reaching solutions that satisfy all parties involved. Active listening and empathy play key roles in conflict resolution. This is particularly important when patients' families are either in a decision-making role (patient is a minor or incapacitated) or when there is conflict among family members as to the best course of action. Utilizing resources such as case managers, clinical social workers, nurse navigators, and the like can mitigate some of the conflicts that may arise from misunderstanding or poor health literacy leading to inappropriate "asks." In situations where conflicts cannot be resolved, engaging an ethics consult may be useful especially in more critical cases where decisions have a significant impact on the patient and the families. Multidisciplinary teams are also extremely helpful in these situations by giving families and all involved providers a range of perspectives to arrive at the best possible decision for the patient.

Confidence and Leadership Skills

Those who communicate effectively are often seen as confident and competent. Strong communication skills are essential for leadership, as they help in persuading, guiding, and inspiring others. In healthcare, this is vitally important as the physician is the leader of the team and guiding the patients' course of action based on the data gathered from history, lab or imaging studies, and the diagnosis. Being able to explain these findings and what the implications of the diagnosis are allows better shared decision-making such that the patient is directly involved in their treatment plan. If the provider seems unsure or cannot clearly articulate the plan, the patients and families can easily lose confidence that they are being cared for appropriately. Even when the diagnosis is unclear or the treatment is uncertain, this can be conveyed in a manner that gives the patient the faith their concerns are being heard, acknowledged, and acted on.

Support Personal Growth and Learning

Being able to communicate effectively enhances learning, whether in an educational setting or through life experiences. It allows individuals to ask questions, seek clarification, and engage in meaningful discussions. Giving patients time to ask questions and think through what was presented to them and allowing them the opportunity to come back at a later setting if needed can really enhance how the encounter is perceived. Providing resources including in some cases referral for a second opinion has been shown to improve the ability for patients to make informed decisions and feel better about how their condition is being managed. Identifying how people relate to communications, be it written, verbal, or video, allows for a better conversation and ability to educate the patients about their health condition and options for management.

Strengthens Decision-Making

Shared decision-making is critically important to engage patients in their healthcare journey. This is a way to ensure buy-in and adherence to care plans, especially in chronic conditions where the patient may be taking medication or undergoing procedures over a period of time. Clear communication aids in gathering relevant information, discussing perspectives, and making informed decisions for all parties. Understanding the patient's perspective may actually alter the care plan based on what the patient is able to do or afford. This then reduces confusion and ensures that all stakeholders are aligned. As was discussed, it is important to ensure who is actually the decision-maker and legally responsible for the patient if they are not capable of making their own healthcare decisions independently. Identifying the legal guardians in cases where an informed consent is necessary is imperative, and if the parent (in the case of the child) is not the legal guardian, having the correct documentation needs to be done before any action should be taken except in cases of emergencies. Obtaining the child's assent in children old enough to understand what is happening also encourages patient participation and more likely to have better adherence to the medical plan.

Conclusion

Effective communication is a crucial skill that impacts every aspect of life. Developing strong verbal, nonverbal, and written communication skills leads to better relationships, career growth, and personal development. Attention should be paid to monitoring the impact of how your communication is being perceived, and working on areas where there may be some miscommunication or implicit biases can pay off over time.

Index

E. Raynor (ed.), *Managing Challenging Patients and Families in Health Care Settings*, https://doi.org/10.1007/978-3-032-10492-2

MIX
Papier aus verantwortungsvollen Quellen
Paper from responsible sources
FSC® C105338

If you have any concerns about our products,
you can contact us on
ProductSafety@springernature.com

In case Publisher is established outside the EU,
the EU authorized representative is:
Springer Nature Customer Service Center GmbH
Europaplatz 3, 69115 Heidelberg, Germany

Printed by Libri Plureos GmbH
in Hamburg, Germany